Keep the Connection

Make the Connection
Ten Steps to a Better Body—And a Better Life
(co-authored with Oprah Winfrey)

Keep the Connection

CHOICES FOR A BETTER BODY
AND A HEALTHIER LIFE

BOB GREENE

HYPERION

NEW YORK

Library of Congress Cataloging-in-Publication Data

Greene, Bob (Bob W.)
Keep the connection : Choices for a better body and
a healthier life / Bob Greene.
    p.   cm.
ISBN : 0-7868-6534-2
1. Physical Fitness. 2. Exercise. 3. Health. I. Title.
GV481.G744 1999
613.7—dc21   99-10484
                                        CIP

PAPERBACK ISBN : 0-7868-8895-4

Hyperion books are available for special promotions and premiums. For
details contact Michael Rentas, Manager, Inventory and
Premium Sales, Hyperion, 77 West 66th Street, 11th floor,
New York, New York 10023, or call 212-456-0133.

Designed by Holly McNeely

Photos by Debra Feingold © 1999

10 9 8 7 6 5 4 3

Acknowledgments

Special thanks to Luchina Fisher, Donna James Robb,
Leila Benjelloun, and the Spa Internazionale at Fisher Island
for their contributions to this work.
In addition, I would like to thank
the many clients with whom I have had
the opportunity to work
for providing entertaining stories
and for being a source of inspiration in my life.

Contents

Preface

In *Make the Connection*, Oprah and I wrote about the steps you would have to take not only to lose weight, but to improve your overall physical and emotional health as well. Those concepts should still form the basis for a healthy way to live your life. *Make the Connection* was a blueprint for getting started and for achieving weight loss. In effect, it was a first step. I know that it helped a lot of people achieve their short-term goals and look at healthy eating and exercise in a new light. But the challenges of lifelong health and fitness are ongoing and require hard work, consistency and patience over your lifetime.

Keep the Connection is a book devoted to those seeking to further elevate themselves physically, mentally and emotionally. It's dedicated to those seeking continual motivation when it comes to their health and well-being. In *Keep the Connection*, I reiterate the things that keep us healthy and fit. I also add some new exercises, including resistance training, that can take you to a new fitness level. And I provide you with nutritional guidance, as well as easy-to-prepare recipes. Above all, I explore the reasons why we lose motivation and offer techniques to keep that motivation intact for the long run. Motivation, after all, forms the foundation for everything we do. Yet it can be so elusive. It seems that either we achieve our goal and lose motivation, or we don't achieve our goal and lose motivation. Regardless, without motivation, permanent change is impossible.

I'm sure you have all heard the saying, "The first step is always the hardest." Personally, I have never cared much for the phrase. Nor do I agree with it. To me, the first step is actually the easiest. Think about it: What are you really risking anyway? If it turns out you weren't ready to take the first step, it's easy to return to your starting point. You haven't stuck your neck out that far.

Or maybe you have taken the steps to achieve your goal, but found that when you reached it, you returned to your "old self." For you, getting motivated is not the problem; sustaining the motivation is.

Taking any kind of action to create positive change in your life is difficult. But the real test happens when you sustain that change over time. That's when you show real strength, discipline and character. **Real change is not made in taking the first step. It's made in the perpetual renewal of your commitment to change.**

Psychologists tell us that most of our behavior patterns are formulated early in life. In other words, we are "hardwired" at a very early age, so to make profound changes as adults involves nothing short of "reprogramming" ourselves. Take for example the person who smokes, has high blood pressure and has elevated cholesterol. The chances are that this person realizes that the three single best things he could do for his health and overall well-being are to stop smoking, get his blood pressure under control and lower his cholesterol. But to give up cigarettes, watch his diet, exercise and perhaps visit his physician occasionally would require him to change behaviors that have been entrenched in his life for years. These behaviors may even act to define him in some way. To make a lasting difference in our lives we have to change not only the choices we make, but the way we think.

In short, real change requires us to transform ourselves.

Keep the Connection

1. Motivation

Since the publication of *Make the Connection* in September 1996, I have had the opportunity to tour the country and speak to thousands of people. After most of these talks, I would spend an hour or two signing books. It became one of my favorite things to do. Once in Duluth, Minnesota, a woman who was waiting near the end of a rather long line asked me, "Do you ever get tired of this?" That had to be the easiest question I'd ever been asked. My answer was an emphatic, "No!" I've always enjoyed answering people's questions about their eating and exercise habits and hearing their personal stories. Quite honestly, I feel like I'm the one who leaves with the most information. I think I learned as much or more in the "signing line" than in all of my years of schooling combined. Mostly, I learned about people.

One important fact I discovered is that people, for the most part, know a great deal about eating right and exercising. They basically know what to do to stay healthy. Let's face it—most of us know that we should eat sensibly and get some regular exercise. It's not a news flash anymore! What people really want to know is how to stay motivated to do these things for the rest of their lives. Without a doubt, it's the number one question I am asked, because without motivation, enduring change is impossible.

You could compare the process of change to renovating your house. If you rebuild your house on a shaky foundation, it may eventually crumble. It's the same with making any change in your body or your health. In the case of your body, the foundation represents the way you think. And self-awareness, self-acceptance, self-esteem and self-love are all the elements that go into building your foundation. They are the same building blocks for motivation. If you want to take this analogy further, you could say that the structure and all the internal workings of the house are fortified by your nutrition and exercise; they keep the house strong and running smoothly. But if your foundation is not solid, your motivation to keep healthy will eventually suffer. That's why the first thing we're going to do in this book is shore up your foundation.

In this section, I will look at the reasons why we lose motivation, how to get it back and ways to maintain it. I'm not going to provide you with gimmicks designed to make you feel better about eating healthy and exercising. I'm going to show you how to get to the heart of who and what you are. It is at this level that true motivation flourishes and real transformation occurs. If you don't know who you are or why you make the decisions you do, then changing the way you behave can be an uphill battle.

All too often, people adopting new health habits underestimate how difficult it will be to stay the course. I'm reminded of this each time people show me their before and after pictures. Of course, I'm happy that they worked hard and found success. Still, I can't help but ask myself, "Will they keep it up? Will they beat the odds?" While they are telling their stories, I find myself listening for certain key words that would lead me to believe they will maintain their success.

You may think this is a cynical view for someone in my field. But, sadly, very few people are able to make permanent changes. The success rate for changing most kinds of behavior is between 5 and 10 percent. Pretty dismal, huh?

Don't worry, we're going to improve those odds. Everything we need to better ourselves—the desire, drive, discipline—we already have. But for many of us, they are buried beneath fear and low self-esteem. That is the reason why changing your body—or anything worthwhile in your life, for that matter—is so difficult. **Poor self-esteem puts you at odds with your own well being.** So to stay truly motivated, you must continually nurture and elevate your self-esteem. Think of self-esteem and motivation as having a symbiotic relationship. If one suffers, so will the other.

Where are you in this process? Are you ready for change? Talking about it, even reading about it, doesn't make you ready. So what is the difference between people who are successful at changing and those who aren't?

After years of working with clients, traveling around the country and meeting people, I began to notice something quite remarkable. In the course of my conversations with people, certain words kept coming up. It didn't matter what part of the country I was in, the same phrases would be repeated time and time again. It got me thinking about the significance of those words. The more I thought about it, the more I realized that people could be divided into three distinct groups based on these words. And these key words were a good indicator of how successful they would be in their efforts to change. The three groups I noticed were the "Yeah . . . buts," the "Whaddya thinks" and the "I loves."

People who continually use the phrase, "Yeah . . . but," feel good in letting you know why they can't change. People who are always asking, "Whaddya think?" are still looking for an external solution to their problem. And people who start their sentences with "I love" are more receptive to improving their lives. While you read about each of these groups, see if you recognize yourself in any of them.

Are you a "Yeah . . . but"?

Linda came to me wanting to lose 25 pounds and improve her cardiovascular health. She had one question, though. "How do I fit exercise into my busy schedule?" It's the second most common question I'm asked, after how to stay motivated. Here is what the usual dialogue with a "Yeah . . . but" sounds like:

"Bob, I really want to lose twenty five pounds, but I don't have the time to fit exercise into my schedule. I have to be at work at eight A.M."

"Well, Linda," I tell her, "if you really want to lose the weight, you're going to have to exercise. And a good workout can take as little as twenty minutes. I'm sure you could free up that much time, especially since you know how much it will improve your health."

"Yeah, I know, but I have a lot to do before I go to work. I have to shower, dress, put on makeup, pack the kids' lunches, get the kids off to school. I would have to get up at six A.M. just to fit everything in."

"That's only twenty or thirty minutes earlier than when you usually wake up. And just look at all the ways it would benefit your life. Come on, you probably hit the snooze alarm three or four times as it is. That's fifteen minutes right there!"

"Okay, you have a point. But I'm not a morning person. The last thing I feel like doing in the morning is exercising."

"If you began exercising in the morning, that would change in about three weeks. You will not only sleep better at night, you'll wake up with more energy. But, if you really don't want to exercise in the morning, what about at lunchtime or in the evening? I'm sure that if you really think about it, you probably could free up some time during the day."

"Yeah, but I'm so tired after work. And lunchtime is out, because there aren't any showers at work."

You get the idea. The key phrase here is "yeah . . . but." If Linda had said it once, I would have thought she was a little resistant to change but still quite capable of doing it. I would have given her an "honorary membership" to the "Yeah . . . but" club. If she had said it twice, I would have thought it was highly unlikely she could make permanent changes in her life—earning her a "charter membership." But three times?! She is now the official poster child of the "Yeah . . . but" club.

You may be thinking that I'm giving up on Linda too easily. Trust me, I've seen many Lindas over the course of 15 years, and she will not find long-term success with her current way of thinking. She is far from permanently changing her life. She's not even willing to make the necessary short-term changes. Forcing Linda to take up a fitness plan at this time would be doing a great disservice to her. It would be setting her up for failure.

Linda needs to spend time reassessing what it is she really wants, how important it is to her, what she is really willing to do to achieve it and whether she is willing to do those things for the rest of her life.

Some years ago, I gave a lecture to a group of health professionals, mostly nurses, exercise physiologists, personal trainers and fitness instructors. I was explaining to them the concept of how some people are just not ready to change their lives. All they really want to do is to *talk* about changing. Essentially, these people want to visualize themselves having a different life, but when it comes right down to it, they are not ready to do the hard work of achieving that life. They are stuck in the "excuse phase." Or, perhaps they are just venting their guilt about not living a certain way.

In my talk, I suggested that, once these people were identified, they were better off working on themselves mentally and emotionally to identify what it is they really wanted—and what they were willing to do to achieve it—before actually making the difficult changes, such as quitting smoking, taking up exercise or altering their eating habits.

To my surprise, the vast majority of the audience was receptive to my point. However, one young exercise physiologist raised an objection. "It sounds like you're giving up on these people," she said. "I was taught that everyone can change and that we shouldn't ever give up. I thought our role is to give encouragement to everyone. I know that's why I went into this field."

It was exactly the comment I was hoping for. Our role, I explained, is to effect change in the most effective manner we can. To push people too aggressively, when they are really not ready to change, is a true injustice to them. Not only will they most likely meet up with failure, but they may ultimately give up on the only thing that can actually help them. I see this all the time when I meet with clients who have been through too many diet and fitness regimens before they were mentally and emotionally ready. They have literally given up on ever trying to change. Their self-esteem has been so battered that it could take months, even years, before they find the motivation to try again.

We are not giving up on these people. We are sending them back home to do their homework! When I finally surrendered blind idealism, I became much more effective in my work. This is especially true in my personal training career. Before I commit to working with a new client, I have about a two-hour initial consultation with them. During that time, if I get one objection ("Yeah . . . but"), a flag goes up. Two or more objections, and I will not work with that client. It may sound brutal, but I've learned that the road to permanent change is tough enough when people appear ready for change. When people place obstacles in front of themselves before even getting started, it's an impossible journey.

Unfortunately, I would say that the majority of people, to some degree, are in the "Yeah . . . but" category. We are all good at coming up with excuses, but the "Yeah . . . buts" are masters. They are trapped in their own excuses. And, for the most part, they feel a bit of satisfaction every time they give you an excuse that confirms to the world that they simply cannot change their life. Inside the mind of every "Yeah . . . but" is someone who would like to live a healthier lifestyle or have the benefits of a healthier lifestyle, but the immediate pleasure and self-validation they get out of defending their current lifestyle is much greater. In effect, they are stuck defending their current way of life.

For some of these people, it's not only difficult but painful to admit that they have made poor choices. It's far easier to defend those choices. And, in many cases, they are not even willing to take responsibility for their choices.

But there is always hope. When people in the "Yeah . . . but" category fully understand the consequences of their current lifestyle and are no longer satisfied defending it, they are ready to change. It will happen when they are all out of excuses and are willing to take responsibility for all of their choices.

If you find that you are a "Yeah . . . but," or have some of these traits, keep reading. There is a wealth of information and mental exercises that will help prepare you for change.

Are you a "Whaddya think?"

The people in the "Whaddya think?" group are second in size only to the "Yeah . . . buts." You can usually recognize them by the use of their opening line; what comes after "Whaddya think?" is as varied as the people in this group are. "Whaddya think?" of . . . the Zone diet, the Atkins diet, the cabbage soup diet, the lettuce diet, high protein diets, zero carbohydrate diets, the jelly bean diet, the chocolate diet, the chewing gum diet, liquid-only diets, the "whatever the flavor of the month" diet; the Thigh Master, the Butt Master, the Ab Roller, the *Buns of Steel* tapes, hand weights, ankle weights, exercise bands, cross-country-ski–trainers, vitamins, chromium picolinate, diet teas, chitosan, Tonalin, Griffonia, 5HTP, fenfluramine, Meridia. . . .

I could go on, but I think you get the idea. Obviously, some people ask me "Whaddya think?" simply because they want to know how I feel about a particular topic, or they may want to incorporate something into their normal, healthy fitness routine. I wouldn't call them bona fide "Whaddya thinkers."

More often than not, however, I encounter the card-carrying members of this group, who are pinning their health and fitness hopes and dreams on, say, popping a miracle pill once in the morning. They are looking for something to take the place of hard work and difficult choices. In other words, they are looking for an easy way out.

I was giving this speech in Southern California, and a man got up to ask me a question. Usually, I limit questions to one or two per person. But this man tried to squeeze in a bunch of questions all at once. He started with "What do you think of high protein–low carbohydrate diets?" I answered, and was about to call on someone else, when he said, "What about chromium picolinate?" After I answered that question, he asked, "Well, do you take a multivitamin?" By his fourth question, the audience began to laugh. "Okay, one more," he said. "What do you think about those Ab-Roller machines?" As I was answering him, it dawned on me what he was doing. He wasn't so much looking for an answer to his questions as he was an answer to the hard work of changing his health: He was hoping to find a substitute for eating healthy and exercising.

Probably the funniest "Whaddya thinker" I encountered was a woman in Memphis. I was signing books after a talk and, again, limiting questions to one or two per person. When it came to this woman's turn, she asked her question. About a half hour later, she showed up at the front of the line again. "Oh, did you think of something else you wanted to ask?" I said to her. She replied, "I had this question before, but I didn't want to be rude to the other people waiting." Twenty-five minutes later, she was standing in front of me again, this time asking me what I thought about something else. Then, as I was about to leave, she followed me to the door while asking me still more questions. Although I appreciated her enthusiasm, I could clearly see that she was looking to me, instead of herself, for the answers.

I'm addressing the entire congregation of "Whaddya thinkers" when I say: There is no easy way. Change requires hard work.

You may argue that at least the "Whaddya thinkers" are thinking about change, which puts them one step ahead of a "Yeah . . . but." Sure, but it's only a small step ahead. When you pin your hopes on a pill, a diet, a piece of exercise equipment, a supplement or the next miracle, you are avoiding the one thing that can really change your life: You. Even people who strictly rely on this book, me or the advice of anyone else are fooling themselves. They still have to do the hard work. My clients discover this when my work with them is complete. Most of them go through an initial period of separation—some will gain weight—before realizing that they were the ones doing the hard work all along. And, they—not me—always had the power to change their own lives.

Stop looking outside yourself for something to change you. Change first takes place inside. This is true in all aspects of your life.

Karen discovered this when she was downsized from her job. For years, she had complained to her friends, family, anyone who would listen, about how much she hated her job. But Karen believed you should never leave your job until you have a better one. She talked to people in her field and sent out her résumé, but none of the jobs she applied for ever seemed right for her. If only she found the right job, she thought, she could leave the city she hated, get a better social life and feel better about herself. Months dragged into years, and still Karen was miserable because she could not find the perfect job. One day, her boss told her the company was cutting back and they would have to let her go, but not without a very generous sever-ance package.

Karen's first thoughts were that her life was over. But after several weeks of being depressed, Karen began thinking about her old childhood dream of becoming a writer. She had the time and the money to try it now, she thought, so why not? As soon as Karen began pursuing her dream, her life changed. She began feeling better about herself, her friends, even the place she lived. Karen still didn't have the job she thought she needed, but it didn't matter anymore. She had changed. She realized that the things she thought a job would give her, she was actually providing for herself.

It really is the same when it comes to improving your health. When you stop looking for the answer outside yourself, you, as a person, can grow. Change is a journey of self-discovery. It's about increasing your self-esteem and feeling better about yourself. If you keep searching for a miracle diet or pill to make all your problems go away, you won't discover anything about yourself. Nor will you increase your self-esteem. And in the end I guaran-tee you won't feel any better about yourself. The only miracle is waiting within you. It will be there as long as you're alive, but now is always the best time to take advantage of it.

If you see any traits in yourself that resemble a devout "Whaddya thinker," read on. There is help for you.

Are you an "I love"?

By far, the smallest of the three groups is the "I loves." It's sometimes hard to find an "I love," but it's always a pleasant experience for me. You know you've found one, when their opening line is "I love," followed by just about anything.

"I love" . . . .the way I feel after my workout, the way I try new things now, walking in the rain, a sunset, a sunrise, the way I feel, the way I feel in the morning, the way I feel all day, the way I feel at night, how I look in my clothes, writing in my journal, meditating, picturing myself reaching my goal, yoga, a good night's sleep, the taste of fruit, traveling, to work out, to cook, to wear hats, to go fishing, to work in my garden. The list is virtually endless.

Who are these people, anyway? They are the people who are done talking about changing their lives. They are either ready to change their lives, receptive to changing their lives, in the process of changing their lives or have already changed their lives. They are willing to make or have already made the connection. They are typically not making excuses, placing obstacles in front of themselves or looking for miracle cures to change their lives. They are taking control. They are doers!

Right about now you may be saying, "Oh, yeah, right. Somebody says they love to wear hats, and this guy thinks they are capable of doing anything." The point is not whether they love to wear hats or walk in the rain; it's that they love *something*. People who use the words "I love" to describe something in their life have a much greater short- and long-term success rate when it comes to getting fit and taking care of themselves.

Here's my theory: When you use the words "I love," you're saying that you feel passionately about something. Passion is the strongest fuel for motivation. Lose passion, and motivation will soon follow. So, at the very least, these people are able to express a seed of passion. This is always a very good sign of future success.

Secondly, people who start a sentence with the words "I love" also appear to have a somewhat positive attitude toward life. An optimist or a glass-half-full kind of person, you might say. A positive attitude is also a powerful predictor of long-term success. In fact, passion and a positive attitude can take you anywhere.

Cecelia has certainly come a long way from where she started. When I first met her, she explained to me that she had gained 65 pounds after a very depressing time in her life, which had culminated in her trying to take her own life. During the first month we worked together, Cecelia had very little enthusiasm or passion for anything in her life. I knew that as long as she remained that way, she would have trouble losing the weight. Sure enough, she had had many setbacks. But her drive and determination saved her. When she returned to her hometown, I found her another trainer, and she continued her workouts. Over the next year, Cecelia and I kept in touch, and I could tell from our conversations that she was changing. Her voice sounded lighter. She laughed more. She was more joyful. Now, Cecelia uses the words "I love" all the time. "I love my dogs," she says. "I love my workouts. And when I don't work out, I feel like I'm missing something. I really love my life."

This remarkable change occurred when Cecelia created a positive cycle in her life through her hard work and determination. This, in turn, made her feel better about herself and her life. To feel good about your life today and where it's going tomorrow is what it's all about.

This is no easy task, especially since we live in a rather cynical time, where feelings of resignation or indifference are all too common. It is much harder to remain positive about yourself and your life. But I believe deep down that everyone wants to be an "I love." That is how we came into the world, but many of us have strayed so far away from it that we have forgotten how to be one.

So how do you acquire passion and a positive attitude? By choosing them. They are choices that you make. So is being motivated. So is everything.

The power of choice

People who create and maintain positive changes in their lives have certain things in common. For one, they invariably have what I call a strong emotional foundation. And the backbone of a strong emotional foundation is self-esteem.

How do we get self-esteem? Are we born with it? Is it something we can acquire? The truth is, self-esteem is acquired early on in our lives, but it requires constant effort on our part if we are to improve and sustain it throughout our lives. The reason self-esteem is so significant is because it's an essential ingredient to effecting change in our lives.

We have the ability to either strengthen or weaken our self-esteem by the choices we make. This is a crucial point. Good choices lead to positive self-esteem, which in turn creates an environment for more good choices. Poor choices lead to negative self-esteem, which in turn creates an environment for more poor choices. In this way, we can create momentum, in either a positive or negative direction, by the choices we make.

Let's use the analogy of a snowball. The more snow you roll it in, the larger it gets. It's the same with self-esteem. The more good choices you pack on, the more positive your self-esteem becomes. And you will want to continue looking for ways to keep the momentum going.

Unfortunately, the reverse is also true. Have you ever had a bad day, where you woke up and didn't feel like exercising? You skipped breakfast, so that by the time lunch came, you ate too much. Then, because you felt bad for overeating, you bought yourself a jelly doughnut for a snack. By the time dinner rolled around, you'd completely given up on yourself, so you ordered a pizza and ate the whole thing, along with a bag of chips, while watching your favorite TV show. The next morning you wake up feeling sorry for yourself and again decide to skip your workout.

I would bet we have all done something similar. That's because when you make bad choices, it's easy to beat yourself up and say to heck with trying to improve. You pack on more bad choices, and pretty soon you've created momentum for negative self-esteem. It can take years to undo this damage. That is why I believe self-improvement should only be undertaken when the person is ready.

It's important to understand how the choices you make affect your life. You are, in essence, what you choose. We don't always realize it, but we are constantly making choices. Life is made up of millions of choices made in every moment of every day of every year in your life. That is how you create who you are—by the choices you make. Look in the mirror. Take a good look at yourself, and understand that you have created this person through all of your decisions throughout your lifetime.

So many people think that to lose weight and get fit, they simply have to alter their choices on diet and exercise. They do. But they also have to take a good, honest look at themselves. And that is probably the most difficult thing to do. You must be willing to look inside yourself to see what needs changing. Then you have to find the strength within to change permanently. In many cases, doing this involves admitting that you have made poor choices in your life. For many of you, this will be a painful admission. It's painful but necessary!

Embracing this concept is essential to accomplishing what you want and, more importantly, keeping what you want. It's a crucial element in the new foundation you're building. As you read on, keep in mind that you create yourself. **You create yourself through choice.**

To understand how, you need to know more about the nature of choices you make in your life.

Making conscious choices

We should always strive to make conscious choices. But because we get in the habit of making certain choices or we are too lazy to think them through, our choices become merely reactions—both automatic and impulsive. Each time the employee is late to work, the boss yells. Every time the little boy falls, his mother comes running. Whenever the woman feels sad, she eats something sweet. If you always react to something the same way, it's a good sign that you need to step back and think before making a choice. You can develop the habit of doing this by practicing what I call the ten-second delay.

The point is not so much to take exactly ten seconds as it is to delay your choice long enough for you to make it conscious. We often make choices in what seems like a split second. I'm asking you to just draw that out a little bit, so that you think before you act. You may find that you make a different choice. But even if you make the same one, you will be more conscious of it.

When it comes to improving your health, there are certain critical moments where the ten-second delay is most valuable. The first is when you get up in the morning and decide whether or not to exercise. Some of you may have already developed the habit of exercising in the morning, because it simply makes you feel better. For you the choice is easy—exercise! Yet others will look at a rainy day or a bad night's sleep as an excuse not to exercise. It's important for them to understand that they made the choice not to exercise. It helps if you tell yourself when you wake up, "I am making the choice to exercise." And if you decide to skip your workout that day, you should tell yourself, "I am making the choice not to exercise." That way you will know that it is up to you.

The same goes for every time you open the refrigerator door or kitchen cabinets to get something to eat. This is another critical moment. If you give yourself a ten-second delay before choosing something to eat, you may not eat it. And even if you do eat it, you will know that it was your choice. A good question to ask yourself while you delay your decision is, "How will I feel afterward?" If you choose to eat a slice of pie, tell yourself what the benefit will be. And if you choose to leave the pie in the refrigerator, tell yourself what benefit that will be. This is a good way to understand the consequences of your choices.

The third critical moment occurs in the supermarket, when you are deciding what should go in your cart. Have you ever returned home, unpacked your groceries and wondered how certain items ended up in the bag? Many times, we go to the supermarket and our minds are somewhere else. Or we go there hungry and let our stomachs do the choosing. The ten-second delay is really an exercise in mindfulness. It forces you to come back to the moment where you are and to think about what you are doing. It can be a tremendous help to you at the supermarket. When you don't allow certain items in your cart, they'll never end up in your home. It's also good to ask yourself why you are buying something. And don't fool yourself into thinking that you're getting it for your partner, spouse or children. If it doesn't fit in with your overall health plan, chances are it won't fit in with theirs, either.

Fear and love: the essence of choice

Entire books have been devoted to what I'm about to condense down to a few paragraphs. For further reading on this and related topics, I recommend the books *A Road Less Traveled* by M. Scott Peck, *A Return to Love* by Marianne Williamson and *The Seat of the Soul* by Gary Zukov.

The main point I want you to understand is that choices are made with the intention of expressing either love or fear. In many cases, we are often unaware of our intentions. That's the first thing we have to change. We have to become more conscious of our choices. I believe if we examined every decision we made, we would be able to determine whether we were driven by fear or love.

Fear is both a gift and a curse. It is essential for our survival. It can protect us and get us out of harm's way. Fear was meant to be primarily a reaction, but it can also be a choice. We are the ones who choose it. Again, we do it out of self-protection. But in some cases, we use it to justify our actions. Or to keep us from feeling pain. Or to distract us from the hard work of change. Or to protect us from the painful thought that we made a mistake and are, therefore, a "bad" person. In essence, we have taken the basic instinct of fear and evolved it into a higher "skill."

There are so many reasons why we use fear to steer our decisions, but the result is always the same: Fear holds us back. And when it comes to realizing our dreams and passions, fear can be a detriment. At the very least, it can delay our dreams. At its worst, it can prevent them from ever materializing.

For some of us, that is exactly what we want, though we may not have admitted it to ourselves. Dreams take hard work. And hard work means constant effort, and constant effort might mean discomfort, pain or, worse, failure. We must protect ourselves from pain, right? So we choose fear. Do you see the cycle?

Remember Karen, who lost her job when her company made cutbacks? She had been making choices out of fear. The reason she stayed at a job she hated for so long was because she was afraid of the alternative. By continuing to search for the perfect job, she could distract herself from having to pursue her true desire: to become a writer.

Perhaps you recognize how you've used fear to make a decision that has held you back. You may wish you could rewrite the past. You can't. But you *can* make a decision now to move toward love and caring for yourself. After Karen lost her job, she could have continued living her life in fear. Instead, she chose to follow something that she loved, and, in doing so, she began making more choices out of love.

Fortunately for us, we were also given the gift of love. Like fear, love can be a reaction or a choice. But a life lived primarily out of love involves effort—much more effort than one lived out of fear. A fearful life is easy. You simply dodge and hide. To live a life of love, you have to be willing to give up fear. That can be a monumental decision. It could mean making huge changes in your life. It could mean giving up your comfort zone and taking some risks. It could involve constant effort.

Have you ever noticed that the people who constantly take risks and live outside their comfort zone tend to have high self-esteem? There is no question that the two are related. While people with low self-esteem appear to be almost manipulated by their fear, people with high self-esteem are more likely to set aside their fear and, more often than not, make choices out of love.

Steve, a guy I met during one of my talks, is doing this now. When I first met him three years ago, however, he was suffering from anorexia nervosa and had to leave law school because of it. Eating disorders are tremendously difficult to overcome. Most of the behavior is driven by fear. To conquer such an affliction, love and caring for oneself must win out over fear. Through reading *Make the Connection*, Steve said he was able to "get a grip" on himself and "realize that there was more to life than dieting." He raised his self-esteem to a level where he began eating better and exercising more reasonably. He returned to school. Now he has a normal body weight and just passed his bar exam. "My future is now wide open," he says.

I like the analogy of life being like a long road with lots of twists and turns. Every so often you reach a fork in the road. Each fork represents a choice. You can choose to follow a path of fear or one of love. If you choose the one leading toward fear, you will need to expend more time and effort to get back to the original fork in the road. This, in itself, is great motivation for choosing the path of love.

Once you put love at the center of your decisions, you are in for a life of constant effort and elevation, constant discipline and evolution—the life we are supposed to live. It's not an easy life, but it's a rewarding one. And the reward is not pain, as is commonly thought. It's joy! A life lived out of love is a life filled with joy.

The connection

I was working out with a client when she asked me if I had finished the sequel to the first book. I told her I was still in the middle of writing it. She then said, "You know, you never defined what 'make the connection' is in the first book. I know what you meant by it, but I'm not sure everyone does. I think you should define it for people."

I began telling her that I wanted readers to interpret the meaning of it themselves. But as I was explaining my decision not to outright define "make the connection," I realized I sounded like a high-school student defending his answer on an essay test. Maybe my client was on to something.

This became more evident as I listened to old radio interviews that raised the same question: "Exactly what does 'make the connection' mean?" I have heard several interpretations, such as the simple, "Oh yeah, that's when you finally 'get it.'" Then there's the more complex interpretation, which I love: "That's when you realize that everything in your life is connected—your health, your relationships, your career, your spirituality, everything. And decisions affecting one area are connected to every other area, as well as your entire life." Both of these interpretations, as well as others I've heard, are valid, but none of them are exactly what I had in mind.

When you "make the connection," you make choices with the intention of expressing love as opposed to fear. That's it. That's the connection: choosing love over fear. The reality is, no one is perfect. It would be unreasonable to think that 100 percent of your choices would be made as an expression of love. This is an ideal to strive toward. You have "made the

17

connection" when you understand this concept and endeavor to make the majority of your life's choices out of an expression of love.

Cecelia and Steve, as well as Karen, have all made the connection. The three of them now tend to make their choices out of love. To get to that point, they each had to first become self-aware. This involves not only knowing who you are, but why you do what you do. Why you react to things in a certain way. What motivates you. What sets you back. Why you have lived a certain way up until now. What your passions are. Your dislikes. In short, understanding yourself involves knowing all there is to know about you.

This may seem like common sense, but it's amazing how few people actually take the time to know themselves. Self-awareness is an ongoing process because we are constantly changing. You can always discover some new insight about yourself, as long as you're open and willing.

In *Make the Connection*, I wrote a section about becoming self-aware. Talking to people, I discovered it struck a chord with many of them and was one of their favorite parts of the book. Because self-awareness is such an important component of a sound emotional foundation, I have included that section and expanded on it here. Some of the recommended exercises may not be for everyone. If any of them cause you extreme emotional pain or discomfort, you may want to seek professional guidance.

Becoming self-aware

All too often, people attempt change without really knowing who they are, what they want or why they really want it. When they end up back where they started, they can't figure out why. If you don't know why you do the things you do, you will keep on doing them. There are some people who aren't even aware of what they're doing. They just know that they keep getting the same results. Yet, they want to change. Without self-awareness, you will stay stuck in the same old rut.

Remember how I said that so many of our decisions are made out of habit or laziness? That's because a lot of us live our lives unconscious of our actions. We are either unwilling or too lazy to take the time to examine our choices and why we make them. Some of us will even put blinders on, because we think it will serve our immediate interests. But in the long run, serving our immediate interests may take us farther away from where we want to go.

To make or keep the connection, you must have self-awareness. Self-awareness is the path toward positive self-esteem. Out of positive self-esteem comes self-acceptance. And when you accept yourself, you experience self-love. Through self-love we learn to love. And to express love is our ultimate goal. That is making the connection.

To live this way is, in itself, a choice. By making that choice, you must be constantly willing to search yourself and your intentions.

Getting to know you

To truly change some aspect of your life—whether it's your health, career or love life—you have to make changes in your behavior. And to do that, you have to know why you behave the way you do. In short, you need to get to know you.

Take the time to understand your strengths and weaknesses, what motivates you, what you like and dislike about yourself, what you can and cannot change about yourself, why you behave a certain way in a certain situation. Do you feel deep down that you have control over your life, or do you feel that you are a victim of life's circumstances? What do you really want out of life? What are your true spiritual beliefs? What makes you happy? What makes you sad? How do you wish to be?

That's what we're going to be doing in this section. We're going to take the time to explore who you are. When I asked people to do the same thing in *Make the Connection*, it presented a challenge for some of them. I'm thinking particularly of one woman who wrote me a letter after the book was published. She said she just couldn't imagine standing naked in front of a mirror and assessing her body. This, to her, would be unbearable.

However, this is exactly what she needs to do, although I realize that it's also one of the hardest things for her to do. I'm sure there are a number of you who can empathize with her. But it was clear to me that this woman was not ready to accept herself. She was unwilling to take a good, hard look at herself, and instead resorted to putting her blinders on. She chose fear. But without ever really seeing or knowing herself, true self-acceptance—and change—will be impossible.

This woman was thinking that if her physical appearance improved, she would feel better about herself and, therefore, would be more receptive to looking at herself. A lot of people feel that way when they first start any self-improvement, but eventually they must come to accept themselves. Without self-acceptance, it's easy to fall victim to the mind-set of: "If only I could lose x number of pounds I would be happy." The problem with this kind of thinking is that you limit yourself to only one of two outcomes. The first is, you never lose the weight and you're never happy. Or you lose the weight and realize that the weight was not the key to your happiness. At that point, you typically start to add on pounds.

Then there is the other extreme—people who are never satisfied with their bodies, who always think they should lose a few pounds, even though they don't need to. For them, body weight and appearance have also become the manifestation for their happiness. Unless they have a perfect body, they can never be happy. It's a catch-22, because achieving a perfect body is impossible.

The key is to accept yourself today. Be happy today, and you will be more likely to do the things that keep you healthy. You will do them out of caring for yourself, out of self-love.

I have also seen instances where clients who have lost a lot of weight will hide or destroy old pictures of themselves. They do this as if to deny that they were ever overweight. In essence, they are denying a part of themselves. I can understand why they may want to put the past behind them. But I think it's more important to remember that we are made up of all the choices we have made over our lifetime and that we should accept all aspects of ourselves, even the painful ones.

To help you get there, I have created some exercises. Just like we have exercises for the body, there are exercises for the mind and spirit. The three work in concert. Remember, you are rebuilding your foundation so your "house" will be stronger. Self-awareness, self-esteem and self-acceptance are crucial lifelong elements.

Exercise 1

The following exercise has helped many people start the important process of improving self-awareness. You will need a journal or a pad of paper, some uninterrupted time and a quiet space.

First, replay your life in your mind. Start as far back as you can remember. Try to recall as many major life events as you can. Pick out three unpleasant events that you most wish you could change. I want you to answer the following questions about each event:

1. When did this event occur in your life?
2. What were the circumstances in your life at that time?
3. Why was this event unpleasant?
4. How did you react to this event?
5. Why did you react that way?
6. How do you wish you had reacted?
7. How would you react today?
8. What has changed in your life since then?
9. What did you learn from this event?
10. When did you learn those things?
11. Did you in any way create that situation?
12. What would you do today in a similar situation?
13. Was there a way to avoid that situation?
14. How did this event change your life?
15. Why do you think this event occurred?

Now recall the three most pleasant events of your life and write them down. Answer the following questions about each of the three events:

1. When did this event occur?
2. What made this event pleasant?
3. Where were you when this event occurred?
4. Who was with you?
5. How did you react?
6. How would you react today?
7. What did you learn from this event?
8. When did you learn it?

Feel free to ask yourself any additional questions. The point of this exercise is to get you to explore your past, to help you begin looking realistically and honestly at your life. It will also help you understand more about yourself; for example, how you react to events. Do you bring these events into your life consciously or unconsciously?

It's important for you to see why events occur in your life. Do they have a purpose? What do they represent? And, most importantly, do you learn from these events? Self-awareness means facing the facts about yourself, both good and bad. Don't cheat yourself. Be completely honest.

Exercise 2

Here's another exercise for self-awareness. It involves your perceptions of yourself. You can do this immediately after Exercise 1, or you can wait a day or so. It's up to you.

1. Describe yourself.
2. Write down three things you like least about yourself.
3. Can you change or improve them?
4. What have you done to change or improve them?
5. How have these things affected your life?

Review your answers, keeping in mind that there are qualities you can change about yourself and some you cannot. But all of them serve a purpose in your life. Each one gives you an opportunity to improve yourself.

6. Write down three traits you like most about yourself.

7. When and how did you acquire these traits?

8. Why do you like them?

9. How has each of these traits affected your life?

10. How has each of these traits given you further opportunities to improve yourself?

11. How has each of these traits contributed to your life?

12. Why do you think you were given these traits?

13. What is their purpose?

Review your answers, and write down any new insights you have about these traits. Since getting to know yourself is a lifetime quest, you should spend time each week or even every day discovering something about yourself. It's always useful to write these things down in your journal. Some other questions you may want to ask yourself are:

What makes you happy?

What makes you sad?

What traits do you like in others?

What traits do you dislike in others?

Are you a patient person?

Are you judgmental?

Are you a hard worker?

Do you have a high or low tolerance to pain?

What brings you pain?

What brings you joy?

What are your spiritual beliefs?

Exercise 3

The purpose of this exercise is to become aware of and take responsibility for your physical self. It helps if you can create a comfortable environment. Now, stand in front of a full-length mirror, either with or without clothes.

The point here is not to shame you, but to give you a true picture of your physical self. This represents a starting point from which you can work. After all, you need to know where you are in order to know where you are going. More importantly, you need to accept who you are right now and take responsibility for your physical self.

To begin

Observe your overall appearance. Take as long as you wish. When you are ready, say these words: "This is where I am today. This represents my life. I could be better. I could be worse."

Next, observe specific details about each area of your body. Start from the top of your head and work your way down. Notice each feature of your face: forehead, eyes, nose, mouth, chin, every detail. Then move to your neck, shoulders, torso and lower body.

Notice those things that you particularly like about yourself. Now notice those things that you don't like about yourself—the ones you can change and those you cannot. Understand that the things you cannot change serve a purpose in your life. Things that you can change are both challenges and opportunities.

Throughout this exercise, keep in mind that the image you see in the mirror reflects not only how you treat yourself—for example, what you eat and how much you exercise—but all the choices you have made to create your life.

In life, nothing stays the same. Your body is no different. It's always changing. And every day, you can choose whether to improve it or let it slide back. This exercise should also help you understand that the choice is yours. Through your choices, you can accomplish whatever you want.

Taking responsibility

When you understand that you create who you are by the choices you make, you are on your way toward taking responsibility for your life—another vital element in building a sound foundation.

We can always point to external reasons for why our lives are the way they are. That's because it's much easier than realizing that we have control over our own lives. Many of my clients would single out their unpleasant childhoods, bad marriages and relationships or unfulfilling careers as the cause for their unhappiness. Their reasons were always external. They projected blame anywhere but on themselves.

Taking responsibility means looking to yourself as the director of your life. It means no longer blaming things outside yourself for who you are. Only when you take full responsibility for yourself and your situation can you begin to accept yourself. And out of self-acceptance comes self-love. Among my clients who successfully changed their lives, all of them at some point let go of all the external causes for their unhappiness with themselves.

I'm not saying you should dismiss certain painful things that happened in your life. We all have events—perhaps from childhood—that have hurt us to varying degrees. Nor am I denying that someone may have seriously wronged you. That person should take responsibility for his or her actions. But to blame people or past events is a waste of time. As adults, we have the power and the ability to deal with those events.

When you take responsibility, you become the cause for action in your life. In other words, you become responsible for transforming yourself. No one else or nothing else does it for you. **You create positive change for yourself by making good, conscious, responsible choices.**

Exercise 4

To look at ways you have taken responsibility in your life in the past, I want you to write down the three best decisions you ever made. Then answer the following questions about each decision:

1. When did you make this decision?
2. Was this a difficult decision?
3. Did you consider any other options?
4. Why do you value this decision?

5. Did your decision come right away, or did you take a lot of time to make it?
6. What would you change about the decision?
7. In what ways did this decision affect your life?
8. How would your life be different if you had made another decision?
9. How did you feel immediately after you made this decision?
10. How do you feel about this decision now?
11. What did you learn from this decision?

Write down what you consider the three poorest decisions you ever made in your life. Then answer the following questions about each decision:

1. When did you make this decision?
2. Was this a difficult decision?
3. Did you consider any other options?
4. Why are you unhappy with this decision?
5. Did your decision come right away, or did you take a lot of time to make it?
6. What would you change about this decision?
7. In what ways did this decision affect your life?
8. How would your life be different if you had made another decision?
9. How did you feel immediately after you made this decision?
10. How did you feel about yourself following this decision?
11. How do you feel about this decision now?
12. Was there anything positive that came out of this decision?
13. If you were given the same situation now, what would be your decision?
14. What did you learn from this decision?

Once you understand the concept of taking responsibility for your life, it's time to ask yourself whether you know what you really want.

Knowing what you want and why

When you don't know what you want, it's often easy to end up somewhere you don't want to be. You're like a balloon, untethered and batted about by the wind. When you have conscious intention, you can set your own course. I'm not saying it will always be a straight road, but at least you'll know where you're headed.

For example, many people who come to me do so because they want to lose weight. But there is always some other, more basic desire beneath their goal. It may be they want to gain self-esteem or the esteem of others. Or perhaps they want to attract someone to their lives or become more attractive to someone already in their lives.

The point is, it's important for you to know exactly what you want. If you want to attract someone into your life, you can do that no matter what size you are. But if you think that losing weight is the only way to do that, you may be setting yourself up for a major disappointment. By putting all your eggs in the losing-weight basket, you ignore other ways to accomplish this goal. And ultimately you place too much pressure on yourself to lose the weight, making the process that much more difficult.

You must understand what your goals represent and why they are important to you. Ultimately, all of our goals represent some form of either giving or receiving love. But it all begins with learning to love yourself.

Exercise 5

This exercise should take place solely in your mind. Later, if you want, you can record your answers in your journal or on a pad of paper. The most important thing is that you believe your responses are obtainable goals. Before you do the exercise, it helps if you can either record the questions on a cassette player or memorize them. This will allow you to keep your eyes closed throughout this exercise.

Start by setting the mood. Turn down the lights, turn on some soothing music, light some candles or incense. Now close your eyes and take a deep breath, followed by a long, slow exhale. After each of your responses,

I want you to take a deep breath, followed by a long, slow exhale. Ready? Now picture a perfect life for yourself.

> What would you look like?
> What would your personality be like?
> How would you treat yourself?
> How would you treat other people in your life?
> What would your relationship with your significant other be like?
> Who would your friends be?
> What types of things would you do with your friends?
> How would you spend the hours in your day?
> What would your hobbies be?
> What would you do for your community?
> What would your spiritual beliefs be?
> How would you express them?
> What would it be like to live this life?
> In what respects is this life different from the one you're leading?
> Why is it different?
> What do you need to do to live this life?

Knowing yourself, taking responsibility for your choices and knowing what you want are the prerequisites for acquiring self-awareness, positive self-esteem, self-acceptance and self-love. These are courses that last a lifetime, since we are always growing and changing.

The choice to change

For some people, the decision to change some aspect of their lives can be quite difficult. In the end, however, it turns out to be the easiest part of the process. It's following through with your commitment that's the most difficult.

Making the choice to change involves not only wishing things were different but also accepting everything you need to do to accomplish the desired goal. This seems so basic, but you would be surprised at how many people underestimate the amount of work that is required to reach their goal.

Exercise 6

It's important to get a handle on exactly what you need to do to accomplish your goals and how that will affect your life. The following exercise may provide a start.

Write down the three most important goals that you want to accomplish in your lifetime. For each goal, record your answers to each of the following questions:

1. Why is this an important goal?
2. Once you reach it, how will your life change?
3. How long do you think it will take to accomplish?
4. Will you need assistance from others to obtain your goal?
5. Write down everything you will need to do to obtain your goal.
6. Write down how doing all of these things will affect your life.
7. Write down all the things you will give up to pursue this goal.
8. Write down one thing that you can do today to help you reach the goal.

Now, do that one thing today that's going to help you reach your goal! If achieving a healthy, strong body is what you want, you will find that it can be one of the best goals for acquiring self-acceptance, self-esteem and self-love. But choose it because it's something you want to do for yourself. Choose it out of love.

The sin of laziness

When we hear the word "laziness," it may conjure up the stereotype of a man reclining on a La-z-Boy, a beer in one hand, the TV remote in the other, when he's supposed to be outside mowing the lawn. Or we may get the image of a woman lying on a couch in the middle of the afternoon, watching soap operas and popping bonbons.

I believe we need to expand our thinking to include a broader inter-pretation of "lazy." Any time you want something or say you want it, and you either don't take the steps to accomplish it or you act in direct opposi-tion to it, you're being lazy. People who complain about their jobs but then do nothing to change the situation are being lazy. Lazy is also when you stay in a relationship even after you know it's not right for you. Or it can sim-ply be avoiding a confrontation with a loved one or friend. It can also be in the form of avoiding the truth, such as not wanting to own up to your past choices. Most of the time, laziness involves some form of fear—for example, fear of an unpleasant consequence, fear of the unknown, fear of success or fear of failure.

It's the same when it comes to your health and fitness. I was at a con-ference recently when a woman came up to me telling me how much she enjoyed reading *Make the Connection* and that she had bought the accom-panying journal. "Did you start writing in it yet?" I asked her.

She replied, "I haven't, but I'm planning on it."

Instead of ending it there, I said, "Well, I find it's always better if you do something today instead of waiting. Like how about walking around the block tonight?"

The woman suddenly looked away. "Oh, I don't know. It's getting dark soon."

I persisted: "Well, how about tomorrow?" She laughed nervously. "I'll do it one of these days," she said.

"The sooner you start, the better," I said. "And it doesn't much matter what you do, as long as you get started."

At this point, the woman looked straight down at the floor. She mum-bled, "Okay."

I touched her arm and told her, "Good luck with everything."

I knew she had an uphill battle. She may have been happy to have found a book that related to her, but she was not really ready to change her life. I've seen many people like her. Deep down they want to be fit and healthy, but they are too afraid to start the difficult process of changing their behavior. They are stuck in the sin of laziness.

When you're being lazy, it's easier to defend your current and past behavior or to come up with excuses for why you can't change than it is to take the steps necessary for change. Not confronting the way you live is a form of laziness. Taking an honest look at yourself and your choices is what this book is about. I don't want you to just read this book and feel better about yourself. I want you to use this book to improve yourself. We can all accomplish more. The ultimate sin of laziness is not trying.

Procrastination goes along with laziness. Procrastination is delaying; it's putting off what you should do today until tomorrow. For most people, tomorrow is never. The woman who came up to me at the conference was procrastinating. Her reply to when she would do something to change her life was "one of these days." When does "one of these days" ever arrive? Procrastination is also driven by some form of fear, not the least of which is the fear of change. It is especially evident among those who struggle with taking better care of their health.

I had just started working with a new client named Bill. He was a high-powered, high-profile executive who owned his own corporation. Bill had neglected his health and fitness for a number of years. His excuse was he wanted to wait until his business was running smoothly. Finally his doctor told him he was headed for a heart attack if he didn't change his diet and get more exercise. Bill hired me and we made a 6:30 P.M. appointment three days a week. From the start, he was late, always citing business obligations as his reason. I knew he was just procrastinating. The first few times, he was 20 minutes late, then he started to be 30 minutes late. Finally I suggested we move the appointment up an hour to 7:30 P.M. "No," he promised, "I'll be there on time." The very next time, he kept me waiting for one hour.

When Bill arrived, he was full of apologies and offered to pay for two sessions. "You are missing the point," I told him, without raising my voice. "Not only are you being disrespectful with my time, you are disrespecting yourself. You made an appointment with me just like you did the people you do business with. Only this appointment should be more important to you, because we're talking about your health here. You are worried about some business meeting when you should be worried about your health. Try buying back your health once it's gone. This should be the most important appointment of your day."

Bill's jaw dropped. I could tell he was not accustomed to being spoken to like that. I was waiting for him to tell me, "Be on your way, trainer boy." Instead, he lowered his head and said, "I'm sorry. It will never happen again." I knew by the tone in his voice that Bill would never be late again, and he wasn't. At first, I thought it was because he had given his word to me, but later I knew it was because he had given his word to himself. He had made a commitment to his health. By making it a priority, he was able to overcome his procrastination and change his life.

Laziness paralyzes us. It keeps us from accomplishing our dreams. It keeps us from facing ourselves and taking responsibility for our choices. It also frees us from ever having to pursue what we really want, and, thus, we never have to face hard work or disappointment.

But once you do take action, even the first step, you can begin to create momentum to counter laziness and procrastination. By taking action, you are initiating a cycle of accomplishment and a desire for more. It's like a snowball gaining size. It happened to Bill. As he became more fit, he saw how his hard work paid off. This was something he had experienced time and again in his business, but never before with his health. The more results he got, the more results he wanted to create.

You can do the same when you make the commitment to something. **Making something a priority in your life is the first step to taking action.**

Exercise 7

This exercise will help you see what you value in life. They are the things that you are committed to. For this exercise, you will need a pencil and paper. First draw a circle at least four inches in diameter. Divide this circle into eight sections, similar to how you would slice a pie. Within each section, write the eight most important areas of your life. Refer to the diagram below for some sample ideas.

Once you have completed the exercise (you do not have to come up with all eight today), draw three lines extending from each section. In each of those three lines, write down three things you can do today to improve that area of your life. Actually being able to see what things are important to you and that you can do something each day to improve them is a great way to keep you motivated and striving for a better life. If you are able to do just one thing each day to improve each area of your life, you will significantly improve your life. If you can do three things each day, at the end of one year you won't be able to recognize your life!

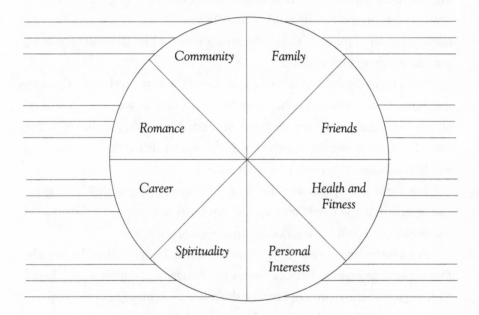

Building a healthy life

Lynn was a vibrant, outgoing executive. She also had struggled with weight her entire adult life. When she came to me, she wanted to lose 40 pounds and become healthier. But as I went through the list of things she would need to do—exercise in the morning, stop eating before 7 P.M. and limit her consumption of alcohol—she gave me reasons why she couldn't do them.

Because she often had staff meetings early in the morning, she couldn't exercise before work began. And since she frequently entertained her clients in the evening, she couldn't possibly stop eating after 7 P.M. And because her boyfriend loved to go out, giving up alcohol was out of the question.

I was hearing a lot of "Yeah . . . buts," yet I still thought Lynn would be successful. "Give me six weeks," I said. "If you still can't handle what I'm asking you to do, then we'll modify it." To Lynn's credit, she said yes, without knowing how she was going to do it. I watched as she overcame every one of her objections. She found she could exercise in the morning by waking up 40 minutes earlier. She moved her dinner meetings to an earlier time, and when the client couldn't meet before 7 P.M., she ate very little or nothing at all. The only thing she thought would be difficult would be completely giving up alcohol.

Lynn had long defined herself as the life of the party and couldn't imagine being that without alcohol. But her greatest fear was that giving up alcohol would mean giving up her boyfriend. Lynn didn't realize it at the time, but deep down she feared that if she wasn't drinking, her boyfriend would think less of her—maybe even leave her.

But Lynn was also committed to following my program for six weeks. We agreed that she would give up alcohol for that time, and at the end of six weeks, she could have an occasional glass of wine.

A lot happened during those six weeks. Lynn dropped about 16 pounds. But, more importantly, her life began to change and improve. She loved working out in the morning, because she felt better throughout the day and got more done. She looked forward to her meals because even the food tasted better to her. And once she realized she was taking care of herself, she wanted to continue. She discovered that an occasional glass of wine was enough for her. She and her boyfriend didn't last, but she even overcame that. As she began feeling better about herself, she began attracting more attention. Lynn was still the life of the party, and she didn't have to give up being healthy to do so. Good health was driving her choices.

When Lynn told me that the weight coming off was great, but finding true happiness was even better, I knew she had made the connection. "I realized I was happy, and it was a gift I hadn't expected," she said. "I always thought my happiness was tied to weight loss. Now, even that doesn't matter as much as doing what's right for me." Lynn has kept the connection for more than a year now. By building changes into her life, she thought she would have to give up a lot. Instead, she gained much more than she ever believed she could.

If you want to change your life, you may have to make some sacrifices. You must be willing to step back and say, "What's the best thing for me?" And if something is not good for you, you have to find the strength to give it up. By giving up certain bad habits, you allow new, healthy ones to form.

Ron was a real estate developer who routinely got to his office by 6 A.M. He had chronic lower back pain that frequently caused him to miss work. He knew that losing weight and exercising would help him, but at first he was unwilling to exercise in the morning. He would also binge after a particularly hectic day. I worked with Ron for four months. He lost 23 pounds and his back problems disappeared. But then he began canceling sessions; before long, he had returned to his old habits and regained the weight. From time to time, I would see him working out on his own or with different trainers, or he would tell me about some new diet he was trying. It was clear that Ron still was not ready to give up his old ways. A year later, I got a call: Ron wanted to know if I would work with him again. He'd given up on gimmicks and trying to find an easy solution to his problems. He now understood that the only way he would improve his health was by changing his life. Life is about trade-offs. But every time you give something up, you gain something else.

You must find a way to meet your goals. Often, change involves subtracting and adding things to your life, and finding a way to make it all work. It takes defining what's important to you, then putting in the hard work and discipline to achieve it. **Once you build change into your life, your life changes.**

Exercise 8

This exercise will help you see how you create your own destiny. Keep in mind that your life is a road with twists and turns and that you will encounter many forks in the road. Recall from Exercise 6 the three most important goals you wanted to accomplish in your life. I want you to write a story about how your life would change if you accomplished those goals. After you finish, I want you to write another story about how your life would look if you didn't accomplish them.

Expecting setbacks and thriving on them

You will encounter setbacks. How do I know that? Because everybody does at some point. The best way to look at setbacks is to see them as challenges. Challenge adds meaning to life. Setbacks really are opportunities for us to grow. If we can overcome them and reach our goals despite them, we have shown true strength, character, discipline and determination. Our sense of accomplishment will be that much greater.

Of course, there are some people who unconsciously wait for setbacks. For them, setbacks become justification for throwing in the towel. It allows them to return to their old habits, their previous way of life—an easier life. If you expect to fail at something, you will look for ways to do that. Don't fall into that trap.

Lynn had a couple of major setbacks when I began training her. We were three weeks into training, and, even though she was working hard and doing everything I told her, she had only lost two pounds. One day, we were in the middle of our stretching, when she asked me what I thought of a diet book called *Sugar Busters!* I told her my opinion. Then, a few days later, she asked me about the modified Atkins diet. After that, it was the Zone. Oh no, I thought, she had become a "Whaddya thinker."

I knew that the real reason Lynn was asking me about these programs was because she had lost only two pounds. She was losing faith in herself. On top of that, she began experiencing knee pain. But she still didn't give up. She switched from running to walking on a treadmill with a steep grade, and on alternate days, she used a stair stepper. With these setbacks, Lynn could have stayed a member of the "Whaddya thinks." Instead, she promised to continue with the program I had set up for her. The following week, Lynn dropped seven more pounds. We now laugh about how she was ready to abandon all her hard work and search for a quick-fix diet program. But the point is, she overcame those setbacks and received a huge boost to her self-esteem.

Temporary setbacks will occur. It's your choice whether to keep them temporary or to make them excuses for why you failed. These challenges can either strengthen your self-esteem or take away from the gains you have already made. It's important to know that setbacks happen naturally whenever you push yourself or try to change your life. They are life's way of asking: "How much do you really want this?" Let's look at some of the more common types of setbacks.

Aches and pains: Aches and pains typically occur when you are pushing yourself to a new level of fitness. We all get them. They are part of training. Training finds your weak link and strengthens it. Most aches and pains are just reminders that you're working hard. However, others are signals to back off slightly.

Sore muscles: If you are doing everything right in your exercise training, you will have sore muscles. They are a by-product of effective training. I always get a kick out of those machines you see advertised on television. The ones that guarantee results without any soreness. That's just not realistic. So get used to a little muscular soreness. When it's difficult for you to, say, walk downstairs, you probably overdid it. For the next few days, work out at a lighter level. Walking or a similar activity that increases your circulation will help alleviate muscular soreness. In most cases, complete inactivity is not advised.

Shinsplints: These, too, are quite common, especially among people who jog, and even more so among those who power walk. Some people are just more prone to shinsplints. But everyone can reduce the odds of developing these inflammations if they warm up and stretch prior to working out. The best stretches for preventing shinsplints are the basic hamstring and quadriceps stretches, as well as those that isolate the calf muscle (gastrocnemius).

If you develop shinsplints, lower the intensity of your exercise until the discomfort is diminished. Also, apply ice to the sensitive areas for 20 minutes two or three times a day. One of those times should be after you exercise. Finally, you may consider taking an anti-inflammatory medication (aspirin, ibuprofen, naproxen) that works for you. If you have never taken an anti-inflammatory or have any other medical concerns, consult your physician.

Blisters: Once I was in the middle of a power walk with a client when she blurted out that she had developed blisters on her feet. "Oh yeah," I said, continuing to walk. "I get those all the time." I didn't see her surprised expression, but I later learned that she thought my remark a little flippant, even insensitive. She had expected me to excuse her from her workout. But there is no reason why most blisters should keep you from exercising. They are simply pockets of water underneath the skin.

The best advice I can give you regarding blisters is to do everything you can to prevent them. Select your athletic shoes based on proper fit—not too tight, not too loose, with adequate room in the toe-box. When you're shopping for new athletic shoes, try them on with the type of socks that you will work out in. They should be made of a special wicking fabric, not cotton, with adequate padding specific to the type of exercise you participate in. If you do get a small blister, place some first aid cream on the blister and wrap it with athletic tape. Replace the tape daily.

For large blisters that hurt, puncture with a sterilized needle and squeeze out the fluid. Use First Aid cream over the affected area and cover with a sterilized gauze pad and athletic tape. If the blister becomes infected, consult your physician.

Injury: Injuries can occur either from your training or from a completely unrelated event. Either way, they can definitely crimp your workouts and your motivation. Any injury should be seen as a signal to care for your body. First, you should always consult your physician for advice. If your physician says it's okay to continue exercising, you can work around your injury. For instance, if you twist an ankle, you might switch from running to either swimming or riding an exercise bike. I have found in many cases that with some slight modification of your workout, you can still get exercise while your injury heals.

Physical fatigue: Usually a temporary situation, it's your body's way of telling you to rest. And you should. After a rest day, you often come back much stronger. This is all part of training.

Mental fatigue: This can be due to your exercise and eating regimen, or to some other aspect of your life. Mental fatigue is frequently a by-product of change, since change introduces a new level of stress—even if it's positive stress—into your life. One form of mental fatigue is simple boredom. Don't worry. This type of fatigue is often temporary. You can sometimes shake it by varying your fitness routine, refocusing on your goals or taking a day off. It may even be a good time to take a vacation. However, should the problem persist, you may want to consult a counselor.

Sickness: Common sense is the rule when you're sick. Obviously, for serious illness, you should consult your physician. For colds and flu, I find that there are always about two to four "bad" days, where you may experience a fever and/or nausea. You should know instinctively when you physically don't feel like exercising, and those are the days you should take off.

Falling short of your goals: For many people, when they don't meet their goals or can't meet them within their designated time frame, motivation quickly evaporates. Quite often, this is a sign that too much emphasis was placed on achieving one specific goal— for example, losing weight. When it comes to achieving and maintaining good health, your goals should be more all-encompassing and ongoing. When you fall short of your goals, set new ones. Remember, it's the entire journey that is most important!

Life hardships: When people encounter personal hardships, such as a death in the family or a job loss, they often relinquish taking care of their health. But that is exactly the time when they should take the most care of themselves. Ignoring your personal health routine during times of hardship will only add to the stress and pain you are feeling. Don't lose sight of yourself or your goals.

Traveling: Sometimes when you leave town, you leave your fitness routine behind. But there is no reason why you can't travel on business or take a vacation and still continue your practice of healthy eating and exercise. You might even plan your vacation around some activity, such as hiking or biking or visiting a spa. Here are a few tips to help you stay focused while you're on the road: always select hotels that have an exercise room; research which restaurants serve healthy foods before you leave; pack your fitness clothes ahead of time; take along healthy snacks.

Living with passion

Without passion, life would become just a series of things we have to do. It would be like punching the clock, putting in our time until we die. What, then, would be the point of doing anything? Without passion, it's easy to become cynical and indifferent and feel like nothing you do matters. A person without passion often feels hopeless, like their life is beyond their control.

A passionate person, on the other hand, can't wait to begin the new day. Each day is filled with the opportunity to do the things you love. And each time you do them, you are filled with zeal and excitement. Remember how I said the people in the "I love" group were passionate about something? That because it's nearly impossible to love something and not feel passion for it.

Passion really is the fuel of motivation. It's what drives us to do the things we love and to do things out of love. When you feel passion for something, it allows you to do the hard work of change. I believe passion was something most of us had in abundance as children. But, as in all things, some of us acquired more of it than others. Can our passion for anything be improved as adults? Absolutely! And one of the best ways to improve it is by caring for yourself. I've seen it happen countless times.

Remember Cecelia? Her goal when she came to me was to lose weight. She persistently worked hard and she saw results. She came to understand that those results were a direct consequence of her efforts. The more effort she put in, the greater the results. It was a wonderful illustration of how she could control her destiny. Once she felt like her life was under her control, it became more meaningful. Her passion for life returned. This, in turn, motivated her to want to continue being healthy.

Karen began experiencing the same thing when she started pursuing her dream of becoming a writer. No longer waiting for a job to change her life, she took her destiny into her own hands. And she began to have real joy for the first time in years. Feeling passionate about what she was doing opened up joy for Karen. Now she's motivated and wants to do other things that will bring her joy.

As you experience passion, it creates a thirst for more. But when you feel like you are stuck in a rut, nothing seems to spark passion. Before Cecelia began changing her eating and exercise habits, she had little enthusiasm for anything in her life. While Karen was in her job, she hated the city where she lived, and was indifferent about her friends and her love life. Passion can bring about powerful results. And results can create a positive cycle of you wanting more—and achieving more—in other areas of your life. For both Cecelia and Karen, passion allowed them to change their lives. Life is no longer about finding ways to avoid pain. It's about living to experience joy!

Often people don't discover this until it's too late. Fortunately, life occasionally gives us little signs that we need to observe. This happened to me while writing this book. I live in a place where I see the cruise ships going out to sea every Sunday. Usually they're gone for a week before returning to port. I'm able to tell them apart by their insignias. There was one insignia that struck me because of its bright colors. It seemed like every time I looked out of my window, I could see it. The fourth time I saw it, I thought, *Wait a minute. Surely, a month hasn't gone by.* But it had. Because I was so preoccupied with my deadline, I was unaware of time passing. And while writing this book filled me with a tremendous sense of joy, I was neglecting my other life's passions. The thought jolted me. I immediately stopped what I was doing, grabbed a good book, hopped in my kayak and rowed out to sea.

Like a lot of people, I occasionally need to remind myself to live in the moment. I used to joke with my clients that my problem was the opposite of theirs. While a lot of them had difficulty delaying gratification, I can delay it into another lifetime! We all need to remember that we only have this lifetime, and we should make the most of it.

The heart patients I've worked with understand this more than most people. A lot of them have faced the prospect of death. Not only are they now more appreciative of life, they are more eager to get on with living it well. I rarely have to worry about finding ways to spark their motivation.

Understanding the limits of time can not only help you break the habit of procrastination, it can also foster passion. And passion fuels the motivation you need to create your life through conscious choice.

2. The Four Components of Fitness

I'm always amazed by the reactions I get whenever I say the words "physical education." The mere mention of this can cause people to groan and grimace. They have a look on their faces that says, "Please, not that again." Most are replaying some horrible childhood memory of being in PE class. Perhaps they are remembering how embarrassed they felt changing into their gym uniforms. Or maybe they are recalling the feeling of never quite measuring up, or the memory of being the last to be chosen for a team. Or maybe they're thinking it was a waste of time—an easy class where all they had to do was show up. It's no surprise that for many of us, our feelings about exercise and fitness are rooted in the way we viewed PE class: as something uncomfortable we're required to do.

In the past, I have tried to avoid using the words "physical education" altogether because of the negative feelings it conjures up for so many people. The more I thought about it, however, the more I realized people were missing the true meaning of physical education; that is, to educate us about how our bodies function and how to keep them strong and trouble-free. That was the purpose of those classes in grade school and high school, even though the message was usually skewed. And that is the point of my job as an exercise physiologist and trainer. Many of us missed that point in school, and it shows up not only in the way we view exercise but the way in which we exercise (or don't). Let's start from scratch. I'll keep this section simple but take the time to read it because by having this knowledge of how your body works, you'll understand why you have to put in the time and effort to achieve the results you want.

First off, it's important to understand that there are different components of fitness. A well-rounded fitness program addresses all of these. All too often, people will either say they have worked out or they have not worked out. They assume that exercise is exercise and pay no attention to the fact that different types of exercises accomplish different goals. Really, there are four components to fitness that we need to be concerned with:

1. Flexibility
2. Cardiovascular power and endurance
3. Abdominal and back fitness
4. Muscular strength and endurance

A good fitness regimen efficiently integrates each of these components. Just so you know, balance and coordination are also considered components of fitness, but since they will typically improve in the course of training the other four, I will not go into detail about them.

Flexibility

Flexibility is the most frequently overlooked component of fitness. It's often the first to get cut from the regimen when time is at a premium. To make matters worse, there are studies that vigorously support the benefits of stretching and studies that claim the results are minimal or nonexistent. No wonder some people are left questioning its effectiveness.

Let me assure you, the time spent stretching will be time well spent. We aren't talking about much time here—about five or ten minutes each day. You might find that it becomes the favorite part of your workout. You may even decide to expand your commitment by stretching longer or adopting a discipline such as yoga. (Not only is yoga great for improving your flexibility, it also builds muscular strength, balance and coordination.) The method of stretching I'll cover here is one of many effective ways to accomplish increased flexibility. The important thing is to stretch!

Understand, too, that we all must work within our given set of genetics. Individuals vary in their level of flexibility just as they do in virtually everything else. The good news is that everyone can improve their level of flexibility.

Flexibility refers to the ability of muscles and joints to give, and thus, allow us to move more freely. As you are probably aware, we lose flexibility in both our muscles and our joints as we age. To an extent, increasing our flexibility allows us to combat some of the effects of age. That's one good reason we should stretch each day. Others include:

- Better performance in athletic or recreational activities
- Less risk of injury
- Reduction in tension and stress levels
- Provides an opportunity to renew ourselves and reflect on our exercise sessions

The technique of stretching has evolved over the years. For instance, a couple of decades ago, stretching was performed ballistically (bouncing up and down), until it began to create as many problems as it solved. A static method then became popular. Using that approach, you hold the stretch anywhere between 15 seconds and two minutes. This static method is still quite common and effective. But I prefer to take it a step further. I want you to hold each stretch for about four seconds, relax for about two seconds, then stretch again for four seconds. Repeat this pattern for about two minutes for each stretch. I consider this the method of choice.

Each fitness expert has a slightly different approach to stretching. There are even different opinions on when is the best time to stretch. You may have heard it's before you exercise, after your workout or both. Personally, I like a little stretching before you begin exercising, but I think it's even more important to stretch *after* your workout. The main point is: *Stretch!*

My personal approach

You should be warmed up before you stretch. When you stretch after your workout, this is already taken care of. But when you stretch before your workout, take whatever exercise you have planned for that day and do it for a few minutes at a lower level. Once warm, you should perform a stretch for each major muscle group using alternating stretching and relaxation phases as follows: Hold each stretch for about four seconds; relax for two seconds; hold again for about four seconds. Perform each stretch for about two minutes. Stretch for five minutes before your exercise session and for about five to ten minutes after your session. Don't bounce. Breathe comfortably while you stretch. Refer to the photos below.

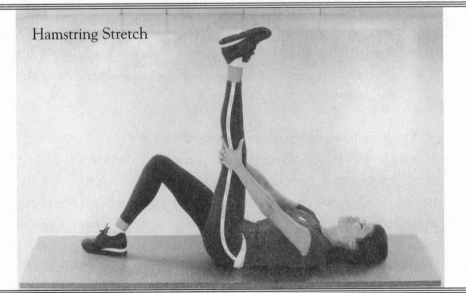

Hamstring Stretch

Hamstring Stretch with Towel

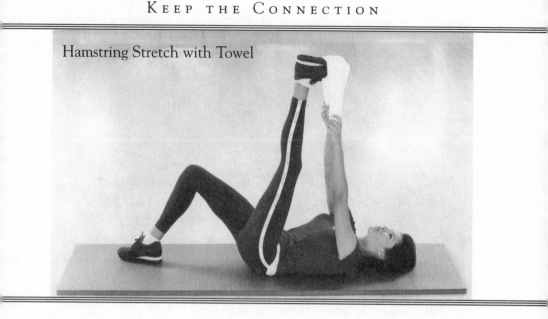

Lie on your back, keeping one leg bent and the corresponding foot on the floor. Raise your other leg up (you can use a towel to assist) until you feel a gentle tension in the hamstring. Repeat on the other side.

Lower Back Stretch

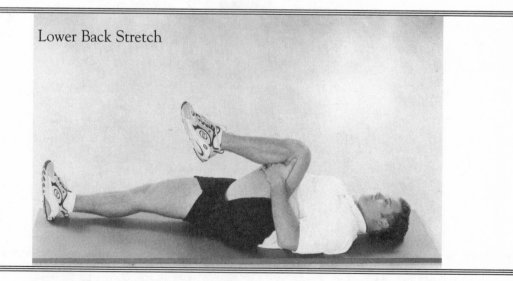

While lying on your back, grab the back of your leg just above the knee. Gently pull that leg toward your chest. Keep your opposite leg straight on the ground. Repeat on the other side.

Buttocks and Lower Back Stretch

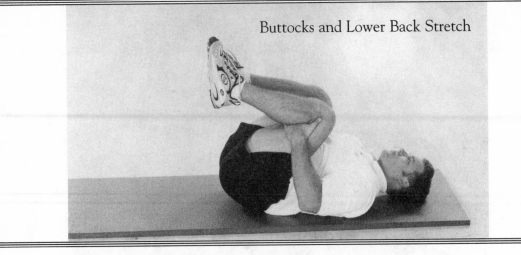

While lying on your back, grab the back of both legs just above the knee and pull them toward your chest.

Inner Thigh Stretch

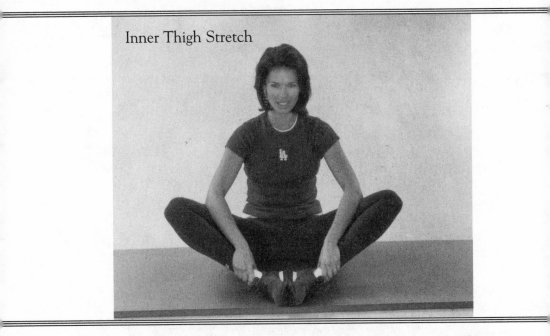

While sitting on the floor, place the soles of your feet together and allow your knees to drop down toward the floor. Gradually pull your feet toward you, until you feel gentle tension in your inner thighs and groin. Lean forward as you become more flexible.

Quadriceps Stretch

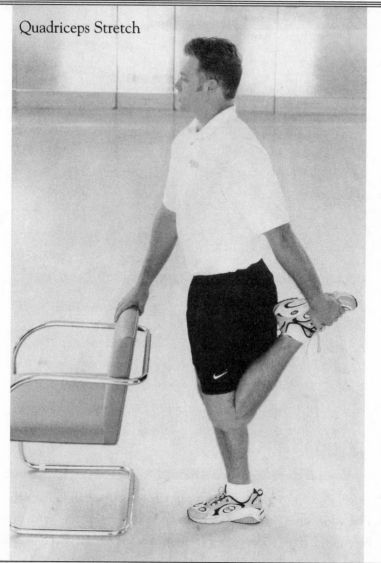

While holding on to something for support, grab your ankle and bend your leg, bringing your heel toward your buttocks until you feel gentle tension in the front of your thigh. The closer you can bring your heel to your buttocks, the more flexible you are. Be sure to keep your knees aligned. Repeat for the other leg.

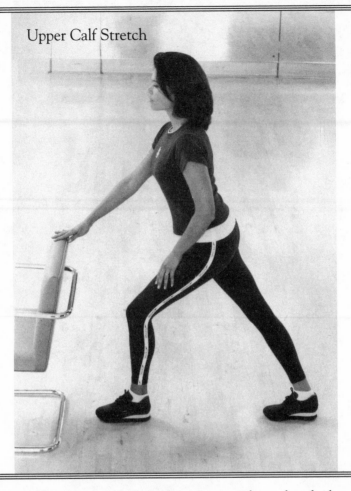

Upper Calf Stretch

While holding on to something for support with one hand, place the other hand on your hip. One leg is kept straight out behind you, with your heel on the ground. The opposite leg is bent in front of you while keeping the knee directly over the corresponding ankle (not ahead of it). The stretch should be felt in the upper calf of the leg that is straight back. If you don't feel it, bring the leg in front (the one that's bent) further forward. Again, you should feel gentle tension. Be sure not to arch your back. Repeat on the other side.

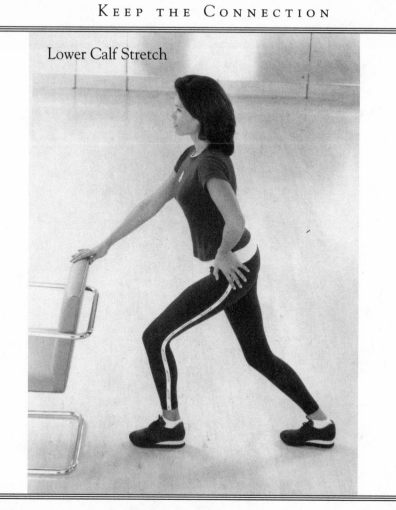

Lower Calf Stretch

While holding on to something for support with one hand, place the other hand on your hip. One foot is ahead of the other and your knees are bent. Bring your hips slowly down toward the floor, keeping both heels on the ground. You should feel gentle tension in your lower calf. Do not arch your back. Repeat on the other side.

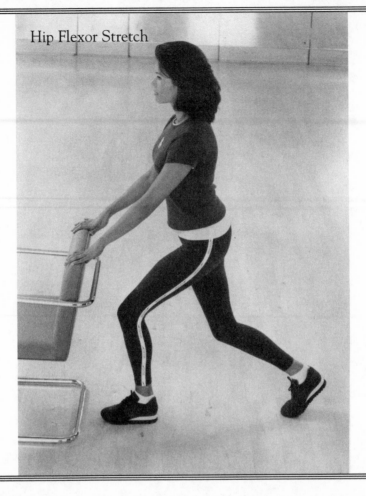

Hip Flexor Stretch

While holding on to something for support with one hand, place the other hand on your hip, keeping your head, neck, shoulders, back and hips aligned. With one leg in front and the other behind, gradually drop in a straight line down toward the floor. Your front knee should be kept in line with your front ankle—not ahead of it. Gentle tension should be felt in the hip of the back leg. You can accentuate the stretch by slightly rolling your hips forward. Repeat on the other side.

Shoulder and Chest Stretch

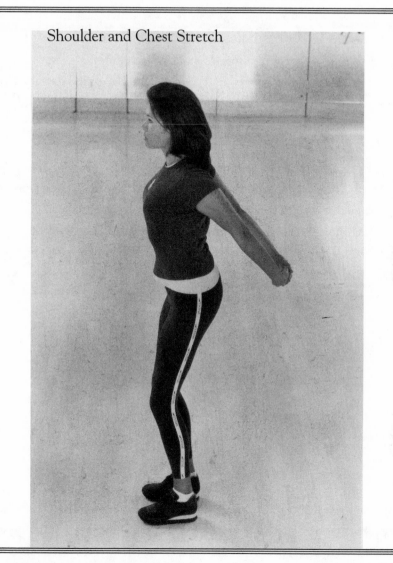

Stand with your head, shoulders and hips aligned and your hands clasped behind you. Your knees should be slightly bent. Bring your hands up toward the ceiling until you feel gentle tension in your shoulders and chest.

The Four Components of Fitness
Cardiovascular power and endurance

Cardiovascular endurance refers to the ability of your heart and lungs to deliver oxygen to working muscles and those muscles' ability to use that oxygen to perform work over extended periods of time. Cardiovascular power simply refers to how quickly your heart and lungs can provide oxygen to the working muscles and how quickly the muscles utilize that oxygen. For our purposes you can consider those terms the same. So when you train your cardiovascular system, you are increasing the body's ability to deliver and process oxygen. **And when you use more oxygen, you burn more calories.** Also in the process of cardiovascular training, the heart and lungs become stronger and healthier. It's no surprise then that our cardiovascular endurance is the foundation of any health and fitness regimen and is therefore a vital component. There are five key elements involved in training your cardiovascular system.

1. Type of exercise
2. Duration of exercise
3. Frequency of exercise
4. Intensity of exercise
5. Progression of exercise

Type of exercise

You may have heard the terms *aerobic* and *anaerobic* exercise. You're probably most familiar with aerobic exercise, but maybe you're wondering what it really means. Aerobic simply means "with oxygen." Exercises that require a lot of oxygen are called "aerobic." They are different from exercises that are "anaerobic," which means "in the absence of oxygen." (The primary energy source required for this exercise is stored in muscle and comes from a process called glycolysis—if you're interested!)

Many people assume that an exercise is either entirely aerobic (such as running or cross-country skiing) or entirely anaerobic (throwing a shot put or weight training). That's really not the case. Virtually every exercise uses energy from your aerobic system as well as your anaerobic system. But different exercises use different amounts of oxygen. When training to improve cardiovascular endurance, our goal is to select exercises that are *primarily* aerobic. When I use the words "cardiovascular" and "aerobic," understand that they are synonymous.

When you train using a highly aerobic exercise, such as power walking or jogging, you increase your aerobic enzymes. Aerobic enzymes will help you burn more fat, so you want a lot of them. In general, the more aerobic an exercise is, the greater effect it will have on your aerobic enzymes and your cardiovascular endurance. Having a strong cardiovascular system will also boost your metabolism, as well as lower your percentage of body fat.

I'll just say a few things about weight training. It is one of the best things you can do for your overall health and to combat the effects of aging. That's why it will be discussed in a subsequent, separate section. But it is a mistake to consider weight training as a method for increasing your cardiovascular endurance. Weight training (or weight lifting) is primarily an anaerobic exercise. To make it more aerobic, the concept of circuit weight training became popular a number of years ago. Circuit weight training involves moving quickly from weight machine to weight machine, usually performing the exercises more rapidly than you normally would. Although this may be slightly more aerobic than traditional weight training, you're not really exercising more aerobically. That's because weight training elevates your heart rate, but it does not use a lot of oxygen when compared to say, jogging, and, consequently, does not increase your aerobic enzymes appreciably. That's why I do not consider circuit weight training an aerobic exercise.

Weight training does, however, have other benefits, mainly increasing and retaining muscle mass, strengthening joints and ligaments and maintaining bone density. I'll cover this topic more thoroughly in the section on muscular strength and endurance.

Choosing an aerobic exercise

You should select a form of aerobic exercise that you feel you have the potential to enjoy. I strongly recommend that you choose a primary exercise, as well as one or two alternate exercises to fulfill the cardiovascular component of your fitness regimen.

Your primary exercise should be one you can readily do—even when you're away from home. It will become the exercise that you are most highly trained in. You should be able to do this exercise about three to four times a week. The alternate exercise(s) you select should be performed intermittently. An alternate exercise will help you tone and train different muscles as well as keep you from getting bored. You'll also be less prone to overuse injuries by choosing more than one exercise.

Your primary exercise must be highly aerobic, relatively easy to perform and convenient. For example, cross-country skiing is highly aerobic, but it's not easy to learn for most people. And outdoor cross-country skiing is not at all convenient, since you need to live where there is constant snow on the ground. One of the main considerations I use in determining the effectiveness of an exercise is whether your weight is supported by you or by a machine (or water, in the case of swimming). When you (not a machine) support most of your own weight, the exercise is most effective from an aerobic standpoint. Of course, this is only a guideline and you can show results with any aerobic exercise. But based on these and other considerations, I have found five exercises that qualify best as primary exercises:

Walking
Jogging
Aerobic dance
Stair stepping (climbing)
Spinning

Walking—Many people don't consider walking to be a great aerobic exercise. It can be, if you do it right. In fact, walking is my top choice for most people. I like it because you don't have to learn a new skill, you don't need any expensive equipment and you can do it just about anywhere. It is highly aerobic when performed properly, yet it does not place a lot of stress on your muscles and joints. In fact, it's one of the only highly aerobic exercises that you can perform each day of the week without great risk of overuse injuries. For all of these reasons, the majority of my clients start out walking. It is, however, still a good idea to add some variety to your routine. Some progress to jogging or aerobic dance; others stick with walking. It's a personal choice.

If you choose walking as your primary exercise, you'll want to be sure you are power walking and not just strolling. There is a distinct difference between the two. To properly perform the technique of aerobic (or power) walking, good posture is essential. It is important to keep your head straight and chin up and to look forward, not down. Keep your shoulders up and level—not hunched or rolled forward. Your hips should be in line with your shoulders, and your back should be erect. Bend your arms at a 90 degree angle and swing them to help propel you as you walk. Make sure that your hands don't reach above shoulder level. And remember, the more you walk, the better your form will become!

Use the checklist below to help you with the technique for aerobic walking:

1. Use good posture
2. Head up, chin straight
3. Shoulders out and aligned with hips
4. Chest out
5. 90 degree arm swing

If you select walking as your primary exercise, you will notice that you become faster as time goes by. This is a sign that good things are happening. You are working harder and you are strengthening your cardiovascular system. I have seen individuals go from a starting pace of more than 26 minutes per mile to under 12 minutes per mile. And always their cardiovascular system becomes stronger as their minutes per mile fall. Start out concentrating on good form, then focus on walking at a level that will bring you results. To help you determine your pace, I'll talk more about intensity later.

Jogging—If you decide to make jogging your primary activity, there are a few things you should know. Jogging typically produces the fastest cardiovascular results, is easy to learn, can be performed just about anywhere and doesn't require a great deal of expense. That's the good news.

The bad news is, jogging places a lot of stress on your body—muscles, ligaments and joints in particular. If you're prone to orthopedic problems, such as strains or sprains of the knee, ankle or hip, jogging may not be for you. In addition, jogging places more stress on your cardiovascular system, which may create a problem for people with high blood pressure or other heart or pulmonary complications. Asthma may present another concern, and if you need to lose a considerable amount of weight, you may have further complications. In these instances, walking is probably a better choice. Your physician or a qualified exercise specialist can help you decide.

The primary difference between walking and jogging is that in walking, one foot is always in contact with the ground. In jogging, you push off the ground with your back leg, so that you are actually airborne for a split second.

Jogging also emphasizes different muscles than walking does. Actually, the two can complement each other well. By using a technique that combines walking *and* jogging, you can get the benefits of both. You simply walk for a while, then jog. When you become tired, return to walking. This is a good technique to use if power walking is no longer producing the desired results and you don't want to jump right into jogging for your entire workout.

Like walking, there is a proper way to jog. For most of us, jogging is a natural activity to perform, and, with consistent participation, we usually adopt good form. Remember to:

1. Use good posture; head up, looking straight ahead
2. Keep shoulders square, slightly ahead of hips
3. Swing arms freely at about a 90 degree angle
4. Let hands hang loosely, move freely
5. Strike the ground with the heel of your foot

Because of the stress to your body, you should only jog a maximum of four times a week. Even when I train people to participate in races, I try to keep their running or jogging to that amount. It is a good idea to combine jogging with an alternate activity to round out your week.

And, as is the case with walking, you should increase your pace according to your ability. Keep in mind that as you become faster, your cardiovascular system is becoming stronger.

Aerobic dance—Aerobic dance—or aerobics—provides what its name implies, a highly aerobic activity. The traditional aerobics class format uses basic dance steps to improve cardiovascular fitness, as well as tone muscles. Today there are many different variations, such as step aerobics, cardiofunk, jazzercise, slide class, water aerobics, even boxing aerobics.

There's no doubt that aerobics classes can offer a fun way to exercise, and, if properly taught, a good workout, too. Even your warm-up, stretching and cool down are built into the class. (I'll say more about the warm-up and cooldown later.) Still, some classes are better than others. For example, water aerobics can be taught as an aerobic activity, but the water prevents your body from heating up as it would in other aerobics classes. Plus, your body weight is supported to a great extent by the water. For those reasons, I don't recommend water aerobics as a primary exercise.

If you choose aerobic dance as your primary exercise, there are some other things you should consider. Soon after the aerobics craze hit, instructors began seeing a lot of overuse injuries in muscles and joints. So lower-impact moves were developed that didn't sacrifice much of the aerobic benefits. Today, most classes are low in impact, even if they are high in intensity. Nevertheless, I believe some injuries can occur if you are taking aerobics classes more than four times a week. I recommend that you do them only three times a week and choose at least one alternate exercise to round out your week. This works well since most aerobics classes in health clubs are scheduled for three days a week.

The best recommendation I can make if you use aerobic dance as your primary exercise is to find a class you like and one that is taught by a qualified, motivating instructor. I recommend that the instructor be certified by ACE (American Council on Exercise) or AFAA (Aerobics and Fitness Association of America).

Stair Stepping—You can perform this exercise on a step machine, by climbing a staircase or by using a set of outdoor steps such as the ones at a stadium. Stair stepping has several pluses. It places little stress on your body; it is relatively easy to learn; and can be an indoor activity, so you're not dependent on the weather.

But stair stepping on a machine is not quite as aerobic as the previous listed activities. That's because when you use a step machine, you are not moving all of your body weight—the stepper supports some of it. You are also using slightly fewer muscles; however, the muscles that are involved do get highly trained.

If you don't have access to a staircase, stair stepping also requires you to either buy a relatively expensive piece of equipment (the cheap steppers are a waste of time!) or to join a health club that has step machines; if you go outside for your stepping, you're at the mercy of the weather.

If you *are* on a machine, it's important to use it correctly. By using the proper form, you can maximize the aerobic benefit of this exercise. All in all, I find stair stepping a great aerobic exercise.

Use the checklist below to help you with your stepping technique:

1. Use good posture
2. Head up, chin straight
3. Shoulders back
4. Hands in contact with machine
5. Arms bent but not supporting entire body weight
6. Take medium to large steps

Keep in mind that you should use your hands for balance, not to support your weight.

Spinning—With the increased popularity of spinning, I have added it to the list of primary aerobic exercises. Spinning is a recent fitness trend that uses a specialized stationary bicycle, music and an instructor in a class format. The instructor takes you on a cycling journey involving varying intensities of cardiovascular exercise. And the entire 50- to 80-minute session is set to music. The popularity of spinning has hit an all time high, for good reason. It can be an exciting way to work out in a group setting. You don't have to learn a bunch of intricate moves or steps as in aerobic dance. And the music gets you moving!

Of course, the excitement of the class is dependent on the instructor as well as the music. Unfortunately, quality classes are not yet available in all areas of the country. Something else to keep in mind. Your weight is fully supported by the bike, which translates into less work, however, this is slightly overcome by the fact that resistance can be added to the wheel.

Alternate Activities

The best choice for your alternate activity would be one of the five exercises just covered: walking, jogging, aerobic dance, stair stepping or spinning. But for more diversity, I have listed some others based on their aerobic potential, ease of learning and convenience. I am not saying these are the only activities you should use, but I think they are the best. They are:

Outdoor cycling
Stationary cycling
Rowing
Cross-country skiing
Swimming

Outdoor Cycling—Outdoor cycling is a moderate to high aerobic activity, depending on how it is performed. But the main reason I recommend it is because it's fun. You can do it with other people or you can use it to get to a destination.

There are a few things to keep in mind, though. First, cycling has a high injury rate from accidents, so it's important to find a route that has minimal traffic. You should also choose a course without a lot of stop signs or traffic lights.

If you cycle as an alternate activity, I recommend that you double the time that you normally exercise. In other words, if you usually stair step for 20 minutes, you will need to cycle for 40 minutes to get the same result. If you have been power-walking for 60 minutes, that means you need to cycle for two hours. You get the idea.

Finally, with cycling, you are at the mercy of the weather. And don't forget to wear your helmet!

Stationary Cycling—Stationary cycling is aerobic enough to be considered an alternate activity. Typically you do not work as hard as you would in a spinning class, but essentially it is the same activity. This activity is also slightly less aerobic than outdoor cycling because there is no wind resistance. Nor are you propelling your weight forward as you do in outdoor cycling. You can partly overcome this by changing the resistance on your stationary cycle.

Among the drawbacks of this exercise: You will again need to double your exercise time to get the same benefit a non–weight supporting exercise, such as walking or jogging, would give you; you might have to buy a stationary bicycle (though there is a device that converts a regular bike to a stationary bicycle); you may also be one of those people who becomes bored by the repetitive motion. On the positive side, stationary cycling is easy to perform; you don't have to worry about the weather; it does not place a lot of stress or pounding on your body; and you can do other things while cycling, such as read or watch television (but don't forget to maintain the proper intensity).

Rowing—Rowing, whether performed inside on a stationary rower or outdoors in a specialized rowing boat or kyack, provides you with an excellent aerobic activity. It places little stress on the joints and ligaments, can be performed indoors or out and conditions both your upper and lower body. If you plan to go outdoors, remember that some boats are better than others. A rowing shell is best for an all-over body workout, whereas in a kayak your arms do most of the work. As for canoes, you are barely using your legs at all. Save it for recreation, after your workout.

If you take up this activity, you may have to buy some equipment and spend some time learning how to properly use it. Also, I should mention that some people find indoor rowing a bit boring.

Cross-Country Skiing—Here's another exercise that can be performed indoors or out. Cross-country skiing is a highly aerobic activity that trains both your arms and legs. There is also little stress placed on the muscles, joints and ligaments. And it is relatively safe—especially on an indoor ski machine.

The disadvantages to cross-country skiing include the cost to outfit yourself. You also have to be moderately fit to participate effectively, and you must learn and practice an intricate skill that requires coordination and balance.

Working out on an indoor ski machine is not as aerobic as skiing outdoors. And you might find it a little boring. On the other hand, to ski outdoors, obviously you'll need enough snow on the ground.

Swimming—I consider swimming a moderately aerobic activity. Overall, it's one of the least stressful exercises for your body, which is why it's an excellent activity to use if you are recovering from an orthopedic injury. Swimming can be pleasant, fun and refreshing. Personally, I love it.

However, there are a couple of drawbacks. The water's cool temperature prevents your body from heating up as much as it would in other activities. This will limit the impact on your metabolism.

It may also increase your appetite. Most triathletes will tell you that on days when they are cycling or running, they won't feel hungry for a few hours. But on swim days, they are ready to eat almost as soon as they leave the pool. Though it hasn't been fully documented, some exercise physiologists, including myself, think that an elevated body temperature actually suppresses your appetite. Just think of when you have a fever; you usually don't feel much like eating. It's the same principle. Unfortunately, swimming does not significantly elevate your body temperature for this to occur.

The other disadvantage to swimming has to do with body fat. The more fat you carry on your body, the more you float and the less you work. That's why, in my first book, I didn't recommend it to people who wanted to lose weight. As a rule, the fitter you are, the more you will benefit from swimming as an aerobic exercise.

A word about recreational sports

You might be wondering about sports, such as racquetball, tennis, handball and basketball. These are for recreation. I don't feel they should be used for a workout session. Each of these sports has active phases and resting phases, and the resting phases break the continuous flow of aerobic activity. By working out, you will be able to participate in these sports at a higher level. So enjoy them, but be sure to get in your workout!

Frequency of exercise

No doubt you have heard conflicting information about how often you should exercise. Only three days a week. Four days a week. A minimum of five days a week. Six days a week with a day of rest. Exercise every day. Feeling confused? I don't blame you. The reason there is so much conflicting information out there is because people are different. They have different abilities, genetics, ailments and, most importantly, goals. In other words, there is no single plan that works for everyone, so each person must decide what's best, based on his or her own needs.

For example, if your goal is to simply live a healthier life and to keep your heart, lungs and circulation strong, three days a week of cardiovascular exercise should do the trick. But if weight loss is your primary goal, a minimum of five days a week is typically needed. In addition, many people need to exercise five, six or seven days a week if they are to remain motivated. For them, a couple of days off can lead to a permanent vacation from their exercise program. In fact, most people do better and are more consistent when exercise is "just part of their normal day." Have I succeeded in completely confusing you?

Let me give you my recommendation for most people: do cardiovascular exercise five or six days a week! When you do this, the health benefits are the most profound—no question about it. You may already be thinking you're going to have to give up everything else in your life to accommodate your exercise routine. Don't worry, you won't. There are creative ways to accomplish everything within a reasonable time frame—based on your goals, of course.

Now that you've digested the fact that you'll be exercising at least five times a week, let's talk about how much time you will need to spend on your aerobic exercise.

Duration of exercise

There is also some confusion about how long you should perform aerobic exercise. We hear that a minimum of 15 minutes does the trick. We hear that we don't burn any fat until after we've been exercising for 20 or 30 minutes. We've heard that low intensity exercise over a long period of time (more than an hour) is best. Again, it all comes down to what it is that you want to accomplish.

In general, you should plan on between 20 and 60 minutes of aerobic exercise per session (preferably five or six days a week). And it is a good idea to vary the length of time: some days do a 20 minute workout; maybe once a week double it or try for an hour-long session if you can. But to really understand why I make this recommendation, you need to know a little bit about how the big picture works. This should help you design a workout plan that is flexible yet effective.

First, it's important to understand the relationship between the duration of your aerobic exercise and the intensity of your aerobic exercise.

(Intensity will be covered in depth in the section that follows.) A number of years ago, it was discovered that people burn more fat by exercising longer at a lower intensity. This lead professionals to prescribe long, slow exercise sessions—especially where weight loss was the primary goal. This philosophy is still sometimes used today. However, to achieve the best aerobic and weight-loss benefits, you need to exercise at a higher intensity. And, to maintain that level of intensity for an entire session, you must typically work out for a shorter amount of time.

The fact that at lower intensities you burn a higher percentage of fat is somewhat irrelevant. I'll say more about that later. The point is, you can, to a degree, juggle the length of time you exercise by adjusting the intensity. You can either shorten the time and increase the intensity or lengthen the time and only slightly lower the intensity. But the key to getting in better shape is being able to maintain your exercise at a **relatively** high intensity for a minimum of 20 minutes. Also, realize that at higher intensities you are more prone to injury—another good reason to keep the workout short.

In general, I prefer shorter (more intense) workouts for most of your weekly sessions to improve aerobic power, and one or two longer, slower (less intense) workout(s) each week to enhance aerobic endurance. A good rule of thumb is, on your long day(s), double your workout time. Obviously this has to fit into your schedule, but this would be optimal. Now let's talk about how hard or intense you will need to work.

Intensity of exercise

Without a doubt, intensity is the most important component of your aerobic workout. The bottom line is, the harder you are capable of aerobically exercising, the better shape you are in. Obviously we don't want to injure ourselves, so we must work within our own individual abilities. For this reason, it's extremely important to learn some basics about exercise intensity.

One of the reasons people believe you should exercise longer and slower is because they've been told it's the best way to burn fat. True, lab tests show that when you exercise at lower levels (50 to 70 percent of your maximum ability), you burn a higher percentage of stored fat versus stored carbohydrates. As you increase your intensity, you begin to burn a higher percentage of stored carbohydrate. This is all true.

So common sense might tell you that since it is fat you want to burn, you should slow down your exercise to below 70 percent of your maximum ability. For those of us who prefer not to exercise at slightly higher intensities—and that's just about all of us—this probably makes a lot of sense. But it's simply wrong.

The truth is, energy is energy. It doesn't much matter what fuel source you burn during your 20 to 60 minutes of exercise. What does matter is safely challenging your body's aerobic power (or cardiovascular power) for about 20 to 60 minutes, which, in turn, will increase your body's ability to provide oxygen to the muscles and the muscles' ability to utilize that oxygen.

The entire premise behind training is to challenge the body and have it respond by getting stronger. Don't challenge it, and little or no change takes place. With low intensity exercise, you are barely challenging the cardiovascular system and, thus, doing little to improve your current level of fitness. Moderately high intensity exercise challenges the aerobic system and increases cardiovascular power. Increase your cardiovascular power and you increase your body's ability to perform work and improve your metabolism. You also decrease your set point and decrease your body fat. In short, you get in better shape.

Even the number of calories you burn during your exercise session becomes somewhat irrelevant. What is important is the rate that you're burning calories both during your exercise session, and the other 23 ½ hours of every day of your life!

Let me put it another way, using my favorite analogy. How many golfers do you know who stroll on the golf course for four or five hours a day, three, four or even five times a week? If they walk instead of ride in a golf cart, they are burning a large amount of calories each round. But I probably don't need to tell you that a lot of these same golfers aren't necessarily in the best of shape. They may easily become winded if they break into a jog.

They may even be lugging a spare tire around the middle. On the other hand, how many runners do you see getting easily winded or carrying around that spare tire? You can bet it's relatively few.

That's because you work harder (more intensely) when you're running than you do when you're strolling the golf course. The intensity is higher. However, strolling the golf course for five hours will burn more calories than 30 minutes of jogging. Again, don't be fooled. Calories burned during your exercise session are not what is important. Challenging your cardio-vascular system is. You do this by working in the zone.

What is the zone?

So, how do you find the zone? In other words, at what intensity should you be exercising to improve your aerobic power?

Exercise intensity has traditionally been expressed as a percentage of your maximum heart rate. I am going to continue expressing it this way so that it's easy to understand, but I'm also going to show you a subjective way to gauge your exercise intensity because I feel this is the way most people should monitor it. I will be asking you to exercise at 70 to 80 percent of your maximum heart rate (7 or 8 on the rating scale). Now let me explain why.

Your heart rate reflects the rate at which your body is using oxygen as well as the rate at which it burns calories (metabolism). The more oxygen your body uses, the more calories you are burning. But remember, it's the *rate* at which you're burning the calories that's important, not so much the total amount of calories you're burning. To estimate this rate of oxygen consumption, we often look at heart rate (the number of heartbeats per minute).

If you have exercised before, you may already be familiar with the phrases "heart rate" and "target heart rate." What you might not know is how we came to use heart rate to measure exercise intensity and some of the problems associated with this method.

Checking your heart rate during exercise is a fair way of measuring how hard you are working. I consider it only fair because there are a number of other factors that can raise your heart rate, such as emotions, thoughts, lifting heavy objects, the environment, even caffeine. Also, you usually need to stop exercising each time you want to know how hard you are working. Nonetheless, exercise professionals have traditionally used the heart rate to monitor exercise intensity. They give you a "target heart rate" based on a percentage of your maximum heart rate. Here's where more of the problems come in.

In order to get your target rate, you have to know what your maximum heart rate is. To get an accurate measurement of your maximum heart rate, you have to take a maximum treadmill test, in which you walk or run until you nearly drop. Sounds fun, huh?

To spare you the expense and inconvenience of the treadmill test, scientists came up with the formula (220 − your age) to estimate your maximum heart rate. To figure out your target heart rate, or the intensity level you should be working at, you have to take a percentage of your maximum heart rate. Usually this percentage is between 50 and 85 percent, depending on the philosophy of the person doing the prescribing.

I must reiterate that I believe that nothing under 70 percent will produce the type of results we are looking for. What I call the "zone" is between 70 and 80 percent. This is the intensity at which I want you to learn to exercise. I also refer to it as the "results zone," because when you exercise consistently at this intensity, you get results. There may be times that you are unable to exercise within this zone. That's all right—sometimes. Exercising at an intensity of 60 to 70 percent is what I call the "maintenance zone." Below 60 percent I refer to as the "almost wasting your time zone." I truly believe that at that level, you will see little or no results. There are some people who exercise at a level between 80 and 90 percent. I don't recommend this for beginning or intermediate exercisers. That's more for highly trained athletes, and even they find it difficult to maintain that level of intensity for an entire exercise session.

Once again, when I refer to the "zone," I am talking about exercising at 70 to 80 percent of your maximum heart rate.

If you find all these numbers and equations confusing and inaccurate, you are not alone. The equation that estimates your maximum heart rate is accurate for only a relatively small percentage of the population. Age, gender and genetics can all skew the numbers.

Once you do figure out your target heart rate, trying to measure it during your workout can be next to impossible. Some of you know from aerobic dance classes how difficult it can be to pause during your workout, locate your pulse and count the number of heartbeats in ten seconds. An estimated 15 percent of all people can't even find their pulse—and I think that's a conservative estimate.

With all this confusion and difficulty in finding your heart rate, I want to suggest another method. First, I want to say that there is no perfect way to monitor exercise intensity. Some people swear by heart-rate monitors. But I prefer a method that requires you to pay closer attention to your body and what's happening to it. What I am about to describe to you is, I believe, the best way to monitor exercise intensity for most people.

A number of years ago, a scientist named Gunnar Borg developed a subjective scale to rate how hard you are exercising. The scale ranged from 6 to 20, and individuals rated how hard they thought they were working. Borg's idea was basically good, but the numbers seemed to confuse people and his descriptions of what each number represented were somewhat vague.

Borg's scale was later modified using a range of 0 to 10. Using these numbers, you rate how hard you are exercising based on your feeling of fatigue. A rating of 0 would mean you were hardly working at all. A rating of 10 would mean all-out exhaustion.

I like this modified scale. But, I've taken it a step further: I have added more detail about how you should feel at each level, with special emphasis on your breathing. I think your breathing is the best indication of how hard you are working.

I use this scale with all my clients, and it works. It may take you a little practice to learn, but it's easy if you are aware of your body and what you're feeling. Very few regular exercisers and highly trained athletes stop to take their pulse to figure out if they are working at their target heart rate. Instead, they become in tune with their bodies and instinctively know how hard they are working. You, too, can learn to feel how hard you're working.

Before I describe this scale, there are a couple of concerns I must mention. You may be in the 10 percent of people who have a hard time subjectively rating your exercise. For you, it's difficult to feel how hard you are working. That's okay. Use the heart rate method. Then there are some of you who may have certain medical problems that would be aggravated if you went above a certain heart rate. You will need to keep track of exactly what your heart rate is doing. Your physician can prescribe a training heart rate for you. You may also use a combination of the two methods to measure it.

Now let's take a look at the scale and the level at which you should be exercising. Some of you may recognize this from *Make the Connection*. I want you to picture a scale from 0 to 10.

|___|___|___|___|___|___|___|___|___|___|
0   1   2   3   4   5   6   7   8   9   10

Rating

0   This is the feeling you have at rest. There is no feeling of fatigue. Your breathing is not at all elevated.

1   This is the feeling you would have working at your desk or reading. There is no feeling of fatigue. Your breathing is not elevated.

2   This is the feeling you would have while getting dressed. There is little or no feeling of fatigue. Your breathing is not elevated. You should rarely experience this low level while exercising.

3   This is the feeling you would have while slowly walking across the room to turn on the television. There is little feeling of fatigue. You may be slightly aware of your breathing, but it is slow and natural. You may experience this right in the beginning of an exercise session.

4   This is the feeling you would have while slowly walking outside. There is a very slight feeling of fatigue. Your breathing is slightly elevated but comfortable. There is a slight feeling of fatigue. You should experience this level during the initial stages of your warm-up.

5   This is the feeling you would have while walking briskly to the store. There is a slight feeling of fatigue. You are aware of your

breathing, which is deeper than in level 4. You should experience this level at the end of your warm-up.

6   This is the feeling you would have when you are walking somewhere and are very late for an appointment. There is a general feeling of fatigue, but you know that you can maintain this level. Your breathing is deep and you are aware of it. You should experience this level in the transition from your warm-up to your exercise session and during the initial phase of learning how to work at level 7 or 8.

7   This is the feeling you would have when you are exercising vigorously. There is a definite feeling of fatigue, but you are quite sure you can maintain this level for the rest of your exercise session. Your breathing is deep and you are definitely aware of it. You can carry on a conversation, but you would probably choose not to. This is the baseline level of exercise that you should maintain in your workout sessions.

8   This is the feeling you would have when you are exercising very vigorously. There is a very definite feeling of fatigue, and if you asked yourself if you could continue for the remainder of your exercise session, you'd think you could, but you're not 100 percent sure. Your breathing is very deep, you can still carry on a conversation, but you don't feel like it. This becomes the feeling you should experience only after you are comfortable reaching a level 7 and are ready for a more intense workout. This is the level that produces rapid results, but you must learn how to maintain it. Exercising at this level is difficult for many people.

9   This is a feeling you would experience if you were exercising very, very vigorously. You would experience a very definite feeling of fatigue and if you asked yourself if you could continue for the remainder of your exercise session, you probably could not. Your breathing is very labored and it would be very difficult to carry on a conversation. This is a feeling you may experience for short periods when trying to achieve a level 8. This is a level that many athletes train at and it is difficult for them. You should not be experi-

encing a level 9 on a routine basis and should slow down when you do.

10 This is the feeling you would experience with all-out exercise. You should not experience a level 10. This level cannot be maintained for very long, and there is no benefit in reaching it.

Take the time to learn each level. Remember, you are striving to achieve a level 7 or 8 during your exercise session. Level 7 equates to approximately 70 percent of your maximum heart rate, while level 8 equals about 80 percent.

Level 7 or 8

Everyone can exercise at a level 7. It may take you a while before you can sustain it for the minimum 20 minutes that I'm asking you to, but you will very quickly work up to it. Remember that when you first exercise at a level 7, you may not like the feeling. This usually goes away within the first month. If you can't keep up a level 7, start at level 6 and step up to a 7 for one or two minutes at a time. Keep extending the amount of time you do this until you are consistently working at a level 7. Usually within a week or two, every client I've worked with has been exercising at a level 7 for at least 20 minutes.

It may be a good idea to exercise with a qualified exercise professional for at least your first couple of sessions. I recommend that this person be certified by either the American College of Sports Medicine (ACSM) or the American Council on Exercise (ACE).

When I first started in the field of exercise science, I was working with heart and pulmonary patients. These were people recovering from heart attacks and heart surgery. They had just been through one of the worst scares of their lives, and my job was to get them healthy and in shape.

A lot of people in my field believed that we should take it easy on these patients, that they should be exercising at much lower levels than everyone else. But watching these patients, I began to notice something. There were some who were comfortable working out at these lower levels and others who pushed themselves to work just a little bit harder. The ones who worked harder showed faster progress—they lost weight, got fit, began eating healthier and stuck to the program I outlined for them. The ones who didn't work as hard saw fewer results, became frustrated and sometimes dropped out of the program.

Clearly, these heart patients were capable of exercising at moderate intensity levels—moderate for them. Perhaps they first started out exercising by walking to the mailbox. But to not push them to work within the zone would have done them a real disservice, because they would be doing little to change their condition.

The same point applies to anyone who wants to improve their body and fitness level. When I began working with weight-loss patients, I noticed that the ones who worked just a little bit harder lost weight faster and had a higher rate of success overall. I also found when I increased the intensity of my own workouts, my fitness level improved significantly. If you push your body to do more, your body will respond by improving. But in pushing your body, safety is always the most important concern. I have spent a lot of time discussing why most people should exercise at at least 70 percent. Also realize that at above 80 percent, you have limited additional gain and much more risk. So stay in the zone!

You may have already figured out that your level 7 will be different from your friend's level 7, or your spouse's or mine. That's why a heart patient can be working at a level 7 and still get the same quality workout as someone who wishes to lose weight or someone training for an athletic event.

Also, you will find that over time, the amount of exercise you can do at a level 7 will change. There may be times that you will want to increase from a level 7 to a level 8 if you want further results. You can also switch to a level 8 for a few minutes in your workout before returning to level 7. This concept is considered interval training. If you are more advanced, you might try working briefly at a level 8.5 or exercising at a level 8 each day.

Now that you've learned about intensity, how do you continue to build on the results of your exercise?

Progression of exercise

A very important component of your exercise regime is your progression—the way you set new goals and accomplish more work. How you advance your performance each day reflects your goals and desires for yourself. In this respect, your progression becomes your philosophy regarding where you want to go. Too many people view exercise as something they to have to do in order to receive some health benefit or desired result. They believe that once they have their "routine" down, all they need to do is show up and punch the exercise time clock. This may work to keep your heart, lungs and circulation healthy and to maintain most of the results that you have so far achieved. But to continue improving your level of fitness, you simply must do more. To fully understand this concept, it helps to know a little about how training works.

When you begin cardiovascular training on a regular basis, you begin to experience results rather quickly in the way of improved aerobic function. But, what causes those results? Let's take a look at your first workout. Obviously you would be performing aerobic exercise at a level above what your body has routinely seen. For example, let's say you begin power walking at a level 7. The muscles, primarily in the legs, need oxygen to perform any kind of work. They will need even more oxygen than normal to perform this new "level" of work. So, the muscles involved send out signals to the heart and lungs that they must provide increased oxygen (which is carried in the blood) to the working muscles. The lungs receive a signal to breathe harder, and the heart receives a signal to beat faster. As a result, more oxygen is presented to the working muscles.

When you begin exercising at a higher level than your body is used to, the working muscles do not have adequate enzymes to process all this additional oxygen. So, to continue walking at level 7, you must provide energy "anerobically." This leads to the production of lactic acid, which, in turn, makes you want to slow down or stop exercising. It also makes you sore for the next few days. The bottom line is, you didn't have enough aerobic enzymes to adequately perform the exercise at that level and/or your heart and lungs could not deliver an ample supply of blood to the muscles. This is a problem, right?

No: This is what happens whenever you are improving and reaching a new, higher fitness level. This is exactly what training is. You should be in the habit of challenging the cardiovascular system on a regular basis if you want to improve. In a sense, what you are really doing during an aerobic training session is starving your body for oxygen. This sends the message to your heart that it must become stronger (similar to what happens to other muscles in our body when we train with weights) and the message to your lungs that they must get stronger and the message to your muscles that they need more aerobic enzymes to process more oxygen. Miraculously, your body responds by strengthening all the necessary systems. It is all contingent on "depriving" (only slightly) the body of oxygen by exercising at an adequate intensity. This occurs most effectively when you exercise five times a week, between 20 and 60 minutes and, most importantly, when you are in the "zone."

You must continue to challenge your body. That is the bottom line of training. That's why if you always walk the same three miles at the same pace, five days a week, your cardiovascular health, as well as your overall fitness and weight, will plateau. Understand that exercise is a stress on your body—a *good* stress! Place this stress on it, to varing degrees, with each workout, and your body will adjust relatively quickly to the demands placed on it. It does so by strengthening itself. In this way, you will always have full control over your own fitness destiny.

Sample progression

Everyone has their own unique genetic makeup, their own exercise likes and dislikes and their own personal goals. It would be impossible, then, to provide a single cardiovascular progression that would be appropriate for everyone. But I think that given the previous information and a sample progression from someone who has begun a walking regimen, you will be able to grasp this important concept and design a progression that is right for you based on your goals. You can apply the same idea to any exercise—jogging, stairstepping, even aerobic dance. The important thing is to have goals and work toward them. It's a good idea to record each exercise session on a workout card or in your journal so that you have a standing record of your progress. It can be a great motivator to actually see your progress. A sample workout card is included after the walking progression.

Sample walking progression

In less than six months, Mary went from walking a mile to doing five miles with weights. It took her a week to two weeks to progress to a new stage of exercise, whereas it might take you or someone else a month. That's okay. You're in charge of your fitness destiny. I've included some samples from Mary's journal to give you an idea of how she progressed.

April 1

I fooled everybody and started walking today. My husband and kids didn't think I could get up at 6 A.M. but I actually did it. I guess I even fooled myself. I didn't feel too bad afterward. It took me about thirty minutes to warm up, stretch, walk a mile and stretch. I actually got to work early and I felt like singing.

April 8

I bought a watch and I'm timing myself now. I can walk a mile in 19 minutes and 30 seconds. Guess I'm ready to move to the next stage: 1.5 miles! Trying to maintain a level 7. It isn't easy.

April 13

I got my first shinsplints. I had to put some ice on my shins. My husband thinks I'm hurting myself. I told him my body is just getting used to being active. I haven't been this active since I was in high school. I already feel that my breathing is easier. Today, I walked 1.5 miles in 28 minutes. I think I'm ready to go a little faster.

April 30

1.5 miles in 17 minutes! I'm almost at half the time it used to take me to walk a mile. Even the runners are starting to notice me now. A few of them smiled at me and said good morning. I guess they see me swinging my arms and sweating like a pig and they know I'm working hard. I feel good, too!

May 10

Wow, so much is happening. I'm walking two miles in under 30 minutes. I guess I'm ready to take on more. I never thought I could feel so good exercising or that I would look forward to doing it every day. On Sundays I don't know what to do with myself, but I know it's a good idea to take at least one day off. Life is beautiful.

May 18

I'm sleeping better, I'm fighting less with my husband, I appreciate my kids more. Something is happening. Could this be the walking? I'm doing 15-minute miles now and I'm up to 2.5 miles. Guess I'm ready for the next stage.

June 1

Everyone is telling me how good I look. I actually went shopping for the first time in months and bought some new clothes. When I tried on my usual size 14 in the dressing room, it was too big. I had to ask the saleswoman to bring me a 12. But even that was too big! I'm actually wearing 10s again. Guess that's what happens when you walk three miles a day.

June 13

I started walking 3.5 miles today. I've been noticing a few more aches and pains than usual, but I think that comes with the territory. I can actually feel my body getting stronger. I'm doing so many things now that I never did before. I've actually become a morning person. I'm happier at work and at home. And nothing gets in the way of my walk. Even when it's raining outside, I still do my walk. I'm also challenging myself more. I want to get down to a 12-minute mile. That's my next goal.

June 22

I'm doing 12-minute miles now. Four miles in 48 minutes!

July 7

My friends and co-workers want to know what my secret is. They can't believe I've dropped down to a size 8 in three months. I keep telling them there is no secret. It's all hard work. I told them, "Six days a week I'm out there first thing in the morning walking four miles while you guys are still snoring away in your beds." But even the way I look now doesn't matter to me as much as the way I feel. For the first time in years, I have real peace of mind. I now understand what it is to live day by day, moment by moment. Walking takes me there. I truly appreciate everything I have.

July 21

I'm doing 4.5 miles now and I think I'm ready to take on more. But I have to decide what it is I want. When I started walking, it was because I wanted to lose weight. I've done that. So now what? I want to improve my tone and strength. I want to start working out with weights. Maybe I should hire a trainer just to help me get started.

Aug. 10

Just finished my five-mile walk. I'm noticing a difference in my body just by using the hand weights one day a week. My trainer wants me to work up to using them three days a week. I definitely feel more tired after my workout, but I think my body will adjust.

Sept. 1

I was just looking back at my journal to the first day I started walking. Wow. I feel like a completely different person. First of all, I never knew I could challenge myself to do so much. Just knowing that I could go from walking one mile in just under 30 minutes to doing five miles in an hour makes me think I can do anything. My husband pointed that out to me the other day when he said, "Mary, you set goals not knowing how you were going to get there, but you did it somehow every time."

Sept. 15

I've decided to stick with walking five miles a day. I'll continue to use the weights three days a week. But basically I'm happy with the way I look and feel. I've decided to take on a new goal. I've always had this dream of having my own business. Tomorrow, I'm going to take the first steps toward starting my own busi-

ness. I know I can do it. Just look at how I've changed my life already. I know the power is within me.

As you can see, your journal is more than just a chronicle of your workouts and how you are progressing. It becomes a record of your dreams and desires, as well as a powerful vehicle for creating change in your life. When you look back at your journal and read earlier entries, as Mary has done, it's easy to see how the things you want can become a reality. If writing in a journal is not for you, a workout card, like the one shown below, can be a helpful record of your progress.

CARDIOVASCULAR WORKOUT CARD

Name _____ Date Started _____
Goals _____ Weight _____
Medical Considerations _____

Exercise	Date						
Walking Treadmill	Level						
	Time						
Walking Outside	Level						
	Time						
Stair Stepping	Level						
	Time						
Aerobic Dance	Level						
	Time						
Spinning	Level						
	Time						
	Level						
	Time						
	Level						
	Time						
	Level						
	Time						

Don't forget to warm up and cool down

It's important to warm up prior to exercising and cool down once you've finished. The warm-up allows your body to gradually adjust to the vigorous workout you are about to perform; the cooldown allows your body to gradually return to its normal state. Note that the warm-up I'm describing here is different from the brief warm-up you should do prior to stretching. Three to five minutes each for the warm-up and the cooldown is usually enough.

Now, I know what you're thinking. It sounds like a lot to do. I'm asking you to warm up prior to stretching, stretch, warm up again, do your exercise, cool down, then stretch again. Well, it is a lot. But after a while, these other things will become part of your routine. They will give you time to mentally prepare, focus and reflect on your workout. In time, you will see how it all only enhances the experience of taking care of your body.

Muscular strength, power and endurance

Muscular strength refers to the muscles' abilty to move resistance. Muscular power refers to the muscles' ability to move resistance quickly. And muscular endurance refers to the muscles' abilty to perform this work for extended periods. They are all important qualities that will be enhanced through the use of resistance (weight) training.

In designing a fitness plan, any one of these qualities can be focused on by either manipulating the number of sets, the number of repetitions, the amount of resistance that is used or the amount of time it takes to move the resistance. You will learn more on this later. For our purposes, understand that all of these qualities will be enhanced in a balanced manner using the techniques described in this section. Also, throughout this section, I will use the terms "resistance training" and "weight training" interchangably. They are essentially the same, but realize that it's not always necessary to use weights to train your muscles. Such is the case with the abdominal–back exercises that I will present later. The exercises shown in this section are primarily for the person beginning a resistance training program. They will improve your overall health, increase your muscular performance, enhance your overall appearance and help you resist the effects of age on your body. If you wish to compete in specialized events or develop a particular area of the body, then you'll need a more in-depth, specialized weight training regimen.

Why should we perform resistance training? The obvious answer to that question would be: to strengthen our bodies so that they function at a higher level and are capable of doing more work. In addition, most people would agree that a strong body is an attractive body. It's also true that maintaining muscle and keeping it active are highly effective ways to control excess weight. These are certainly nice benefits of resistance training, but I believe the most important one is combating the effects of age. Two of the most profound effects of the aging process are the loss of muscle and the loss of bone (osteoporosis). Resistance training is the best way to fight both. This is not a theory, a hunch or an opinion. It is just plain fact. Your time spent resistance training is time well spent.

First, you must understand that your resistance training is an entirely different activity than your cardiovascular workout. Many people make the mistake of trying to make them interchangeble. They are not. They accomplish very different goals. The five days of aerobic exercise each week are optimal for training your cardiovascular system. The three days a week that you should be training with weights are over and above that. These two different activities can be performed within the same workout sessions, but, again, they cannot be substituted.

There is at least one similarity between the two. If you want to show improvement, you must continue to challenge yourself. Just as with aerobic training, there are various factors essential to an effective resistance training regimen. They are:

1. Repetitions
2. Sets
3. Amount of resistance (weight) used
4. Time increment between sets
5. Frequency
6. Progression

7. Types of Exercises:

  Abdominal–back exercises

  The basic eight weight training exercises

Repetitions—Repetitions refer to the amount of times you overcome a resistance (lift a weight) prior to taking a break or resting. As I mentioned earlier, weight training builds muscular strength, power and endurance. And the number of repetitions and the amount of weight used can dictate which of those qualities is stressed. In general, a higher number of repetitions (using a relatively low amount of resistance) builds more muscular endurance, whereas lower repetitions (using a relatively higher weight) builds muscular strength. Performing the exercise more quickly will help build muscular power, but that's not something I will stress in this book, since most of us will not be competing in the shot put in the upcoming Olympics. In addition, lifting for power (lifting quickly) is a technique that has a higher risk of injury with little benefit to the average person. For our purposes, the resistance, or weight, should take from two to four seconds to lift. And each repetition should be performed immediately after one another.

To maximize the benefits of resistance training, I recommend that you have between eight and ten repetitions in each set. For training the abdomen, where no resistance other than your own body weight is used, I like to use repetitions of 15. This will nicely complement and benefit your regular cardiovascular exercise. I also want you to select a weight that you can lift between eight and ten times, so that at the final repetition the primary muscles involved will be fatigued. By fatigued, I mean you should feel a slight burning in the major muscle group involved in that exercise and that lifting any further repetitions would be very difficult.

Sets—A set refers to a grouping of repetitions of the same exercise. For example, you can do a "set" of crunches, a "set" of bench presses, a "set" of leg extensions. You get the picture. The entire premise for weight training is that you fatigue the muscles and they respond by getting stronger (and/or gaining endurance). Doing multiple sets enhances fatigue, which, in turn, enhances the training effect. If you are just beginning to perform weight training, it's a good idea to start with only one set for each exercise and eventually build up to a maximum of three sets. Keep in mind that when multiple sets are added, you may not be able to lift the same number of repetitions as in the previous set. This is actually desired because when this happens, you know that the muscle is being fatigued and that training is taking place. Many current programs of resisitance training use only one set of a particular exercise. While research shows that improvement takes place using one set, I still like to train most people to eventually use either two or three sets. I feel that multiple-set training adds another dimension to the training processs and is well worth the extra effort. I'll go into this in more detail in the section on progression.

Amount of resistance (weight) used—Selecting the amount of resistance you use should obviously be based on your individual capabilities as well as your goals. Traditionally, trainers, when initially setting up your program, prescribe a resistance between 60 and 80 percent of your maximum, with 70 percent being the most common prescription. To arrive at this number, often a maximum lift is performed and the prescribed percentage calculated. This is an acceptable method, but I personally prefer another. Start with a very light resistance and, through trial and error, arrive at a weight that, as described above, makes you fatigued after lifting it eight or ten times. Prior to each set in your normal routine, a warm-up set should be performed. The warm up consists of four or five repetitions using about half of your prescribed resistence. This will warm the muscles involved in the lift and minimize the risk of injury. When you are capable of doing multiple sets, start your next set following a short 15- to 30-second rest interval.

Time increment between sets (rest interval)—One of the most common errors associated with resistance training is that too much time takes place between sets. Obviously this applies only to those who are doing multiple sets. This rest interval between your sets is a critical training element and should be respected if you want to maximize your workout. All too often I see people daydreaming or having conversations in between sets. This is not only a less effective way to train, it is also holding up everyone else's workout while they wait for the equipment. The main reason people take too much time between sets is because it makes resistance training easier. The more time the muscles get to recover, the easier it is to do the next set of repititions. But it is much better to have a shorter rest interval and not be able to complete the number of repetitions in your next set. As a matter of fact, that's exactly the desired effect. You know good training is taking place if you cannot complete as many repetitions on your second set as you could on your first and fewer still if you do a third set.

How long between sets should your rest interval be? It should be 15 to 30 seconds for the basic eight exercises and about five seconds or the amount of time to take one deep breath for the abdominal–back exercises. When you first start with the basic eight, 30 seconds between sets is recommended. The more conditioned you become, the less time you will need in between sets. If you are currently resistance training, try shortening the time between your sets. You will notice it's much harder. But it won't take you long to get used to it. Not only will you show better results, your workouts will shorten considerably.

Frequency.—Resistance training as infrequently as once a week will maintain your current level of muscular strength/endurance. Slight improvements can be seen when you up the frequency to two times a week. But for most people, I recommend resistance training three times a week for the basic eight exercises and six or seven times a week for the abdominal–back exercises. This will give you an optimal level of improvement with a minimum time investment.

Progression—How aggressively you advance your resistance training is strictly a function of what you want to accomplish and how hard you want to work. Safety and injury prevention should be your primary consideration. There are, however, certain cues that will tell you when you are capable of doing more work. The following progression is a good one for the majority of people.

First, I believe that the abdomen–back area is the single most important muscle group to train because it stabilizes the entire body and is almost always involved whenever we lift anything. Strong abdominal and back muscles are a major influence on our posture as well. The successful training of all of the other muscle groups relies on strong abdominal muscles in particular. That's why I like for my clients to do abdominal–back exercises for at least one month prior to training with weights. I recommend the same to you. Start your resistance training by performing the routine outlined in the section on the abdomen–back. After about a month of training the abdomen and back, or when you feel you are strong enough, start the rest of your resistance program by doing one set of all the basic eight exercises outlined in the back of this section.

If you are setting your weights properly and working hard you will notice a slight soreness in the muscles that are exercised. This is not only normal but desired. However, if the soreness is uncomfortable to the point where you don't feel like training, the weights are probably set too high and should be lowered. There will come a time when you notice that the same routine using the same resistance no longer produces any muscle soreness and you feel like you could do several more repetitions without a problem. That's a good time to add a second set to each exercise—again, using the same weights as before. When the second set becomes easy to the point where you could do 12 or 13 repetitions relatively easily, it's time to add your third set. Remember, you should be resting only 15 to 30 seconds between sets.

When you have progressed to three sets of all eight exercises, you can further your results by adding more resistance. You may need a little trial and error to find the exact weight you should be lifting. Again, use a resistance that fatigues you after eight or ten repetitions. Whenever you notice that you can lift the current weight more than ten times, you can decide to increase the weight. However, you should do this in the smallest increments possible for safety's sake and to see how your body responds. One final way to progress your program is to use a shorter rest interval between sets, but you should keep it within the 15- to 30-second guidelines. Now, your progression is completely under your control and influenced by your individual goals. Keeping a record of your repetitions, sets, weights, exercises and progression not only helps you organize your workout, it's a good motivational tool as well. A sample workout record is shown at the back of this section.

Types of exercises

Abdominal-back exercises—Even though the abdominal muscles and the muscles of the lower back are separate muscle groups, for our purposes I will refer to the exercises in this section as abdomen-back exercises since they both serve the important function of stabilizing the torso. As mentioned before, one of the most important muscle groups, and often the most overlooked, is the abdomen. The abdomen, as well as the back, form the center of your musculoskeletal system; any time you lift anything, your abdomen and back act to stabilize your body.

Many people are under the false impression that doing abdominal exercises will reduce the amount of fat in the abdominal region. Unfortunately, there is no such thing as spot reducing—much to the dismay of all the manufacturers of those devices designed to reduce fat in a given area and to the people who have purchased them. For our purposes, the abdominal-back area should be viewed as a unique muscle group and should be trained differently than the other muscles.

The abdominal area is actually a grouping of muscles. To maximize this area's potential, you must train using different exercises with different positions. I don't particularly care for the abdominal machines that have become so popular since they train at a fixed angle. Also, those devices claim to protect the neck by resting it on a pad, but they are actually preventing the neck from getting stronger. In fact, the neck is extremely weak in most people who do not train using abdominal crunches. Yes, the neck is vulnerable to injury during training, which is why it's important to train the abdomen and neck together.

There are two philosophies when it comes to doing crunches. One has you roll your head forward and place your chin on your chest. The other has you keep your head straight. Each method has its own strengths and weaknesses, and either is acceptable. All things considered, I prefer the latter method for most people. Keep your head straight with your chin pointed toward the ceiling as you go up. When you first start performing these exercises, you should place your hands gently behind your neck for support. But do not roll the neck. As you get stronger, you can move your hands to rest on your collarbones.

The rules for training the abdomen and back are slightly different from training the other muscle groups. The abdomen–back is the only muscle group I recommend you train every day or at least almost every day. I use 15 as opposed to eight or ten when training the abdominal–back group. The reason I do this is because these muscles support our bodies all day long, making the quality of muscular endurance especially important. In addition, the rest interval between sets is shorter—about the amount of time to take a deep breath. And as I said before, make sure your abdomen is strong before you begin resistance training the other major muscle groups. Typically a month of abdomen–back exercises is adequate.

When you take a look at the exercises, you'll notice they are called crunches and not sit-ups. A number of years ago, sit-ups were used to strengthen the abdomen. Then it was discovered that the traditional sit-up placed unnessessary stress on the back. Also, by fully raising the torso, the hip flexor muscles can become tight, exacerbating some people's back problems. Now, we do similar exercises called crunches. But the torso is raised only about 30 to 45 degrees off the floor, and the knees are always bent, with the exception of the leg-up crunch and the arm-leg raise.

Now let's take a look at the abdominal–back exercises. Keep in mind that the following exercises are not intended for those with serious back problems. In addition, these exercises may not be appropriate for individuals with neck conditions or high blood pressure. If any of the following exercises cause pain or discomfort other than that associated with normal muscular strengthening, discontinue their use and consult your physician. As always, you should consult your physician before performing any new exercises. The recommended abdominal–back exercises are listed below:

- Basic crunch
- Twisting trunk curl crunch
- Knees to the side
- Legs at 90 degrees
- Vertical legs crunch
- Extended arm crunch
- Reverse trunk curl
- Arm-leg raise

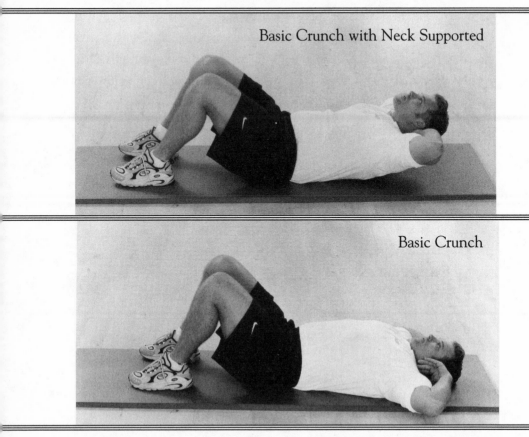

Basic Crunch with Neck Supported

Basic Crunch

Bend your knees, keeping your feet flat on the floor, and place your heels 12 to 15 inches from the buttocks. Place your hands lightly behind your neck. As your neck is strengthened, you may rest your hands lightly on your collarbone. Use your abdominal muscles to raise your torso off the floor. Your chin should go straight up toward the ceiling with no flexion (rolling) of the neck. Be sure to keep your shoulders square. Raise your torso up to a 30- to 45-degree angle. Pause for a split second before returning to the starting position. Do not hold your breath during any exercise. Continue until the set of 15 is complete. Take a deep breath and begin your next set.

Twisting Trunk Curl Crunch with Neck Supported

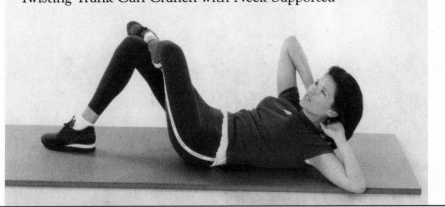

Bend your knees and place your heels 12 to 15 inches from the buttocks as in the photo above. Then place your right ankle on your left knee. Place your hands lightly behind your neck. As your neck becomes stronger, you may rest your hands lightly on your collarbone. Use your abdominal muscles to raise your left shoulder up toward your right knee (your right shoulder should only be off of the floor between 8 to 12 inches). Pause for a split second at the top and return to the floor. Be sure to use your left arm, which is resting on the floor, as a fulcrum (or pivot point). Continue until the set of 15 is complete. Take a deep breath and begin your next set. When you are finished doing the number of sets you chose for yourself, switch to the other side so that your left ankle is on your right knee. Repeat the set(s) on this side.

Knees to the Side Crunch with Neck Supported

Knees to the Side Crunch

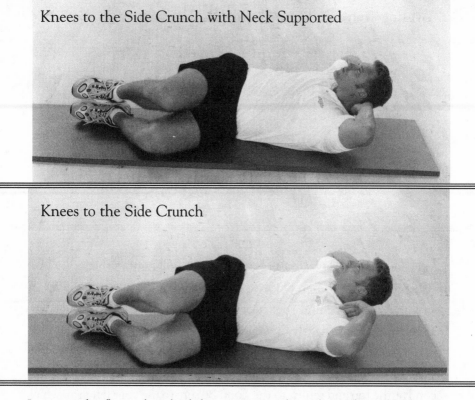

Lying on the floor, place both knees over to the right as shown in the picture below. Now make your shoulders square. Place your hands lightly behind your neck. As your neck becomes stronger, you may rest your hands lightly on your collarbone. Use your abdominal muscles to raise your torso off the floor. Your chin should go straight up toward the ceiling with no flexion (rolling) of the neck. Be sure to keep your shoulders square throughout the crunch. Your shoulders should come up only two to four inches off the floor. You should feel this exercise at the extreme side of the abdomen on the opposite side that your knees are on. Continue until the set of 15 is complete. You may have to build up to 15. Take a deep breath and begin your next set. When you complete the number of sets you have chosen, switch your knees over to the other side and repeat the set(s).

Individuals who have back conditions should avoid this exercise or consult their physician before performing it.

Legs at 90 Degrees Crunch with Neck Supported and
Legs Supported

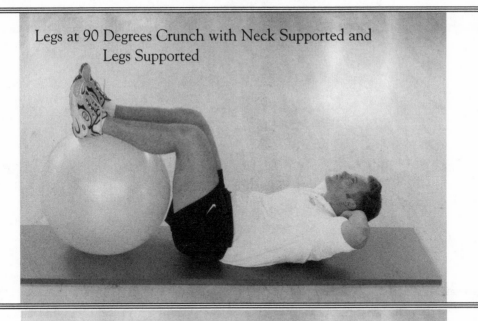

Legs at 90 Degrees Crunch with Neck Supported

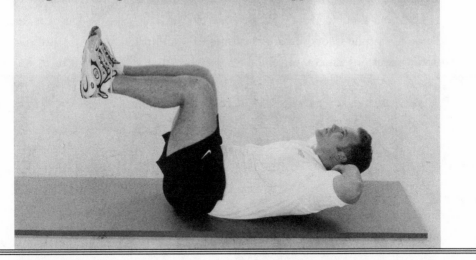

Your legs should be off the floor and bent at the knees at a 90-degree angle. It's a good idea to support your legs with a chair, exercise ball or place your feet on the wall until you are strong enough to hold at the 90-degree angle on your own. Place your hands lightly behind your neck. As your neck is strengthened, you may rest them lightly on your collarbone. Use your

Legs at 90 Degrees Crunch

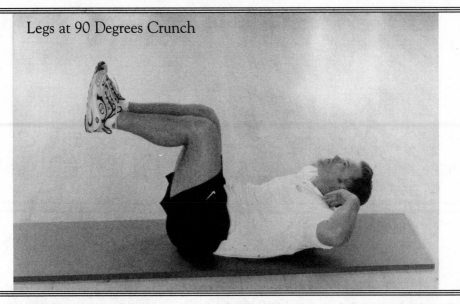

abdominal muscles to raise your torso off the floor. Your chin should go straight up toward the ceiling with no flexion (rolling) of the neck. Be sure to keep your shoulders square. Raise your torso up to a 30- to 45-degree angle. Pause for a split second before returning to the starting position. Continue until the set of 15 is complete. Take a deep breath and begin your next set.

Vertical Leg Crunch with Neck Suported

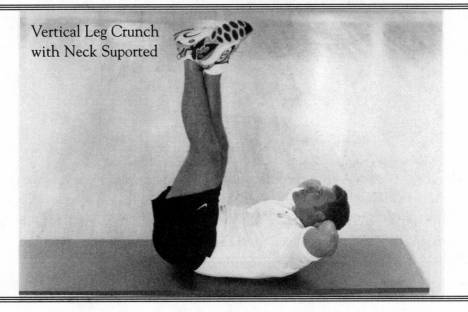

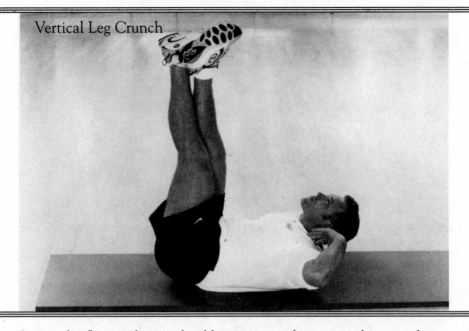

Vertical Leg Crunch

Lie on the floor with your shoulders square and raise your legs straight up so that they are perpendicular to the floor (90 degrees). Place your hands lightly behind your neck. As your neck is strengthened, you may rest your hands lightly on your collarbone. Use your abdominal muscles to raise your torso off the floor. Your chin should go straight up toward the ceiling with no flexion (rolling) of the neck. Be sure to keep your shoulders square. You should raise your torso up to a 30- to 45-degree angle. Pause for a split second before returning to the starting position. Continue until the set of 15 is complete. Take a deep breath and begin your next set.

Extended Arm Crunch with Neck Supported

Extended Arm Crunch

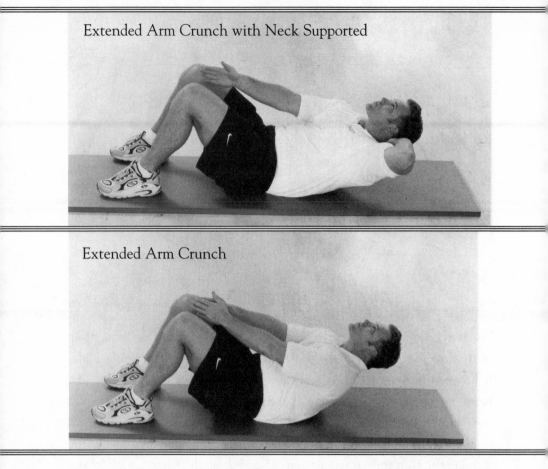

Bend your knees, keeping your feet flat on the floor, and place your heels 12 to 15 inches from the buttocks. Place one hand behind your neck for support. Extend the other arm straight out so that it is between your knees. As your neck is strengthened, both arms can be extended straight out. Use your abdominal muscles to raise your torso off the floor. Your chin should go straight up toward the ceiling with no flexion (rolling) of the neck. Be sure to keep your shoulders square. You should raise your torso up to a 30- to 45-degree angle. Pause for a split second before returning to the starting position. Continue until the set of 15 repetitions is complete. Take a deep breath and begin your next set.

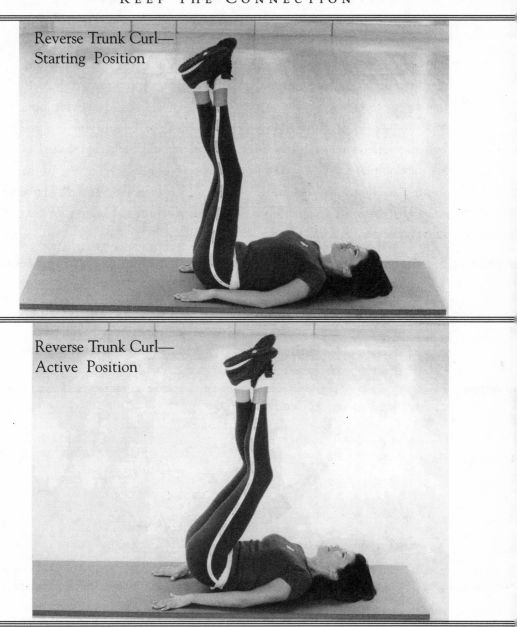

Reverse Trunk Curl—
Starting Position

Reverse Trunk Curl—
Active Position

Lie on your back with your legs straight up at 90 degrees, knees slightly bent. Keep your hands palms down by your sides. Your back should remain on the floor as well as your shoulder blades. Contract your abdominal muscles first, then curl your pelvis up making your feet go up toward the ceiling. Begin to exhale upon contraction of your abdominal muscles. Your hips should rise only three to five inches off the floor. Be sure your legs and buttocks remain relaxed—the primary work should be accomplished by your abdominal muscles. Pause for a split second before returning to the starting position. Continue until the set of 15 is complete. You may have to build up to doing 15 repetitions. Take a deep breath and begin your next set. This one takes some practice!

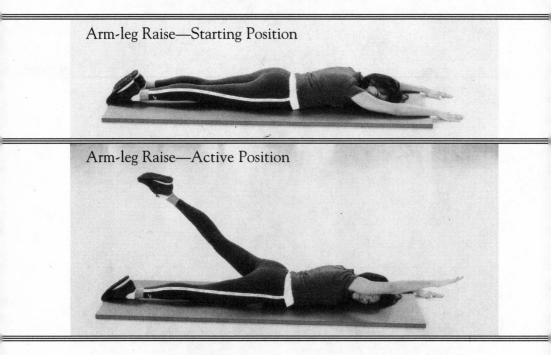

Arm-leg Raise—Starting Position

Arm-leg Raise—Active Position

Lie face down on the floor with your head turned to the left and your arms extended over your head. First, contract the abdominal muscles and the muscles of the lower back. Then, raise your left arm and your right leg simultaneously. Keep your shoulders and your pelvis pressed against the floor. Do not lift your arm and leg too far—you should lift until you feel gentle tension in your lower back muscles, then return your arm and leg to the floor. Exhale on the way up and inhale on the way down. Continue until the set of 15 repetitions is complete. You may have to build up to 15 repetitions. Take a deep breath and begin your next set. When you have completed your chosen number of sets, switch to the other side, lifting your right arm and left leg. Repeat the set(s) on this side.

The basic eight resistance exercises

When combined with the abdominal–back exercises, the basic eight exercises listed below work all the major muscle groups of the body. Keep in mind that there are different types of equipment and different techniques that can be used to perform each exercise. I realize that you must use whatever equipment you have access to; and while some is preferred to others, a good resistance program can be built using a variety of equipment and facilities. My personal recommendation: Go to a gym, as opposed to your home, if you can. Not only will you find all the equipment you need (and help using it), but exercising outside the home can give you a much-needed mental break from everything else in your life.

The most important thing to remember is to practice safety and proper form when doing these exercises. That way you can be sure that you are adequately training all of the major muscle groups. The following instructions and photos represent the exercises well, but nothing can replace having a knowledgeable instructor or trainer take you through each exercise. Working out with a trainer is no longer a luxury for just a select few. It's a little-known fact that you can employ a trainer for just one session to plan your workout and take you through each exercise. You can even have your trainer outline a year's progression for you. It's well worth the one-time fee. Should you decide to try it, I recommend finding a trainer who is certified by either the American College of Sports Medicine (ACSM) or the American Council on Exercise (ACE).

Before you start each lift, don't forget to warm up using four or five lifts with about half the resistance.

THE BASIC EIGHT:

Leg Press
Leg Extension
Leg Curl
Chest Press
Bicep Curl
Tricep Extension
Shoulder Press
Upright Row

Primary muscles involved:
Buttocks, Quadriceps, Hamstrings

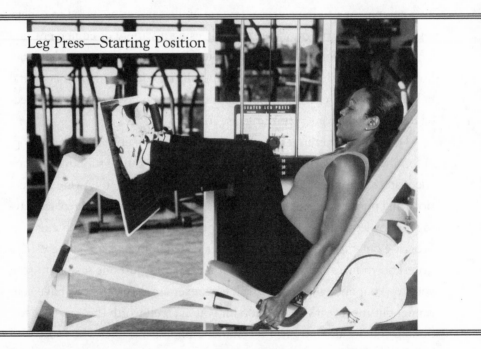

Leg Press—Starting Position

Starting position Select a seat setting that allows you to fully extend your legs. The body should be erect with the back firmly against the seat. The feet should be squared or turned slightly outward, with the weight on the ball of the foot. Your legs should be flexed at 90 degrees or less when starting the exercise.

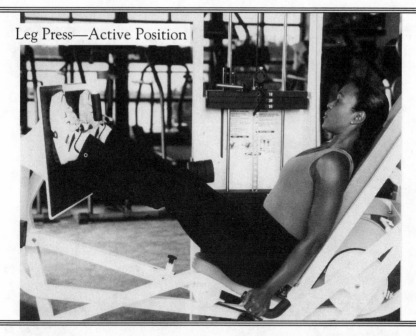

Leg Press—Active Position

Active phase Prior to lifting the weight, contract your abdominal muscles. Extend your legs completely when lifting the weight, but do not lock your knees. Exhale on the extension phase. Pause for a split second before returning the weight to the starting position, inhaling on the way back. The extension should take two to three seconds, as should the return. After completing each repetition, pause for a split second before starting the next repetition. Continue until the set of eight to ten repetitions is complete. Take a deep breath, wait 15 to 30 seconds and begin your next set.

Common Errors

- Seat adjusted improperly: either too close or too far from the weight
- Leaning forward; back is away from the pad
- Dropping the weights back to the starting position too quickly
- Not breathing during the exercise
- Not tightening abdominal muscles prior to lifting the weight
- Locking the knees at full extension

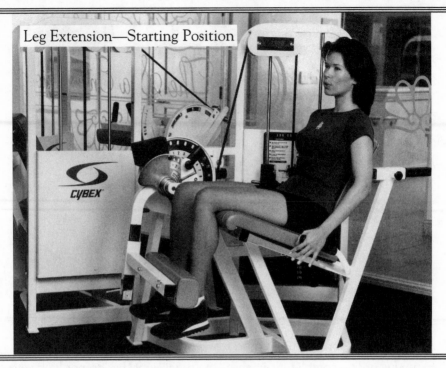

Leg Extension—Starting Position

Primary muscles involved:
Quadriceps

Starting position Adjust the leg arm of the machine so that your knees are centered with the pivot point. The leg pad should be adjusted so that it rests comfortably above the feet. The body should be erect with the back firmly against the seat. Grasp the handholds firmly and look straight ahead. Your toes should be pointed straight up or with a slight pitch inward. Your legs should be flexed at 90 degrees when starting the exercise. Your thighs should be parallel to each other with about four to five inches of space between your knees.

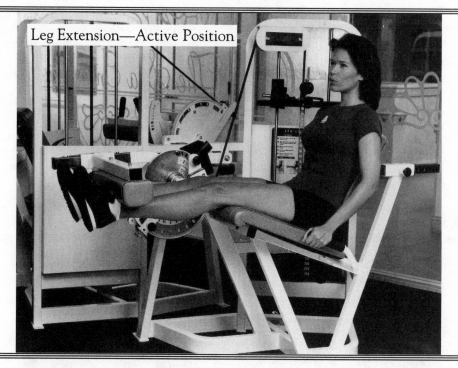

Leg Extension—Active Position

Active phase Contract your abdominal muscles before lifting the weight. To lift, extend your legs completely without locking your knees. Exhale on the extension phase. Pause for a split second before returning the weight to the starting position, inhaling on the way back. The extension should take two to three seconds, as should the return to the starting position. When each repetition is complete, pause for a split second and start the next repetition. Continue until the set of eight to ten repetitions is complete. Take a deep breath, wait 15 to 30 seconds and begin your next set.

Common Errors

- Poor posture: shoulders rounded; head down
- Allowing the back to lift off back pad
- Lifting too much weight
- Lifting the buttocks off the seat while lifting the weight
- Kicking the weights up instead of lifting them slowly

- Not breathing during the exercise
- Not tightening abdominal muscles before lifting the weight
- Placing hands on legs instead of the hand grips
- Dropping the weight quickly to the starting position instead of lowering it slowly

The photo below shows a seated leg curl machine. There is another machine that has you lie face down on your abdomen while curling the weight toward your buttocks. I strongly recommend the seated leg curl because it takes a lot of pressure off your back, reducing the risk of injury.

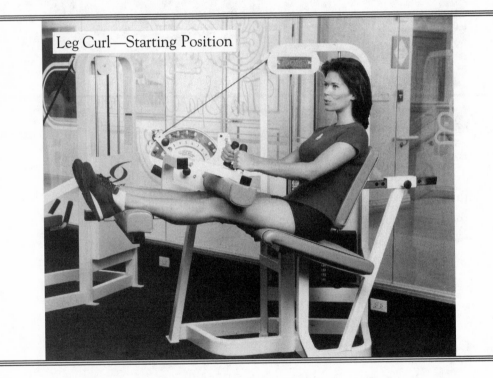

Leg Curl—Starting Position

Primary muscles involved:

Hamstrings

Starting position Adjust the leg arm of the machine so that your knees are centered with the pivot point. The leg pad should be adjusted so that it rests comfortably on the back of the leg, just above the achilles tendon. Lower the thigh stabilization pad to fit snugly across the thighs. The body should be erect with the back firmly against the seat. Grasp the handholds firmly. Your toes should be pointed straight up or with a slight pitch inward. You should be looking straight ahead. Your thighs should be parallel to each other with about four to five inches of space between your knees. Your legs should be straight but not locked.

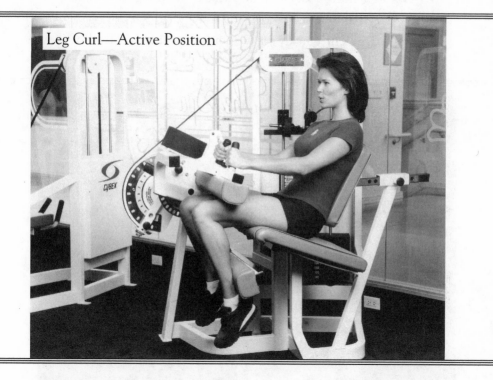

Leg Curl—Active Position

Active phase Contract your abdominal muscles before lifting the weight. To lift, move your legs down to a 90-degree angle. Exhale on the beginning of the downward phase, then pause for a split second before returning the weight to the starting position, inhaling on the way back. The downward phase should take two to three seconds, as should the return to the starting position. When each repetition is complete, pause for a split second and start the next repetition. Continue until the set of eight to ten repetitions is complete. Take a deep breath, wait 15 to 30 seconds and begin your next set.

Common Errors

- Poor posture: shoulders rounded; head down
- Allowing the back to lift off back pad
- Lifting too much weight
- Raising the weights up too quickly instead of controlling them
- Not breathing during the exercise
- Not tightening abdominal muscles before lifting the weight
- Placing hands on legs as opposed to hand grips
- Raising weight quickly to the starting position instead of slowly controlling it

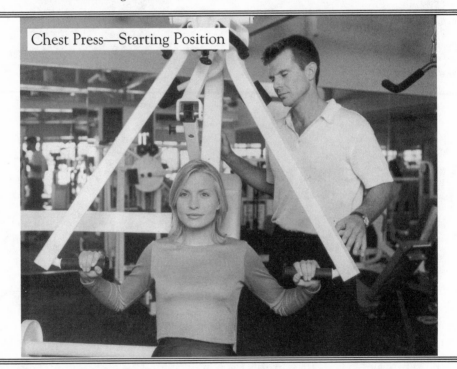

Chest Press—Starting Position

Primary muscles involved:
Chest and Triceps

Starting position Adjust the seat height so that the handles are at the middle of your chest. The body should be erect, with the back firmly against the seat. Grasp the handholds firmly, with your hands positioned approximately four to six inches in front of your chest. Your upper arms should be parallel with the ground. Position your elbows slightly below the handles.

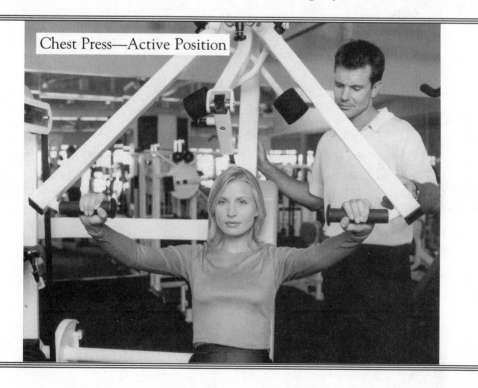

Chest Press—Active Position

Active phase Contract your abdominal muscles before lifting the weight. Begin the lift by pushing the handles forward with a smooth controlled movement. Be sure to exhale on the extension phase. And keep your shoulder blades pinched together and your elbows at handle level throughout each repetition. Pause for a split second before returning the weight to the starting position, inhaling as you do so. The extension phase should take two to three seconds, as should the return to the starting position. When each repetition is complete, pause for a split second and start the next repetition. Continue until the set of eight to ten repetitions is complete. Take a deep breath, wait 15 to 30 seconds and begin your next set.

Common Errors

- Poor posture: shoulders rounded; head down
- Allowing the back to lift off of back pad
- Lifting too much weight
- Improper adjustment of the seat
- Not breathing during the exercise
- Not tightening abdominal muscles before lifting the weight
- Not performing the lift with full range of motion
- Performing the initial phase of the exercise too quickly
- Returning the weight to the starting position too quickly instead of slowly controlling it

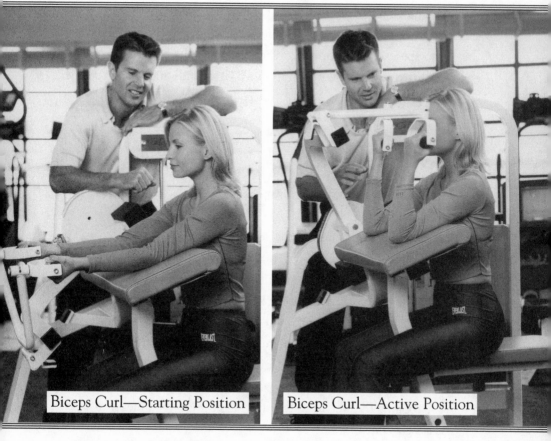

Biceps Curl—Starting Position

Biceps Curl—Active Position

Primary muscles involved:
Biceps and Upper Arm

Starting position Adjust the seat height so that your elbows are slightly lower than your shoulders when seated. Rest your chest against the pad. Place your elbows on the pad and centered with the axis on the cam of the moving arm. Grasp the handholds with an underhand grip.

Active phase Contract your abdominal muscles before lifting the weight. Curl the weight upward as far as possible. Be sure to control the movement. Return to the starting position gradually. Exhale while lifting the weight up, inhale on the return to the starting position. The initial lifting phase should take two to three seconds, as should the return to the starting position. When each repetition is complete, pause for a split second and start the next repetition. Continue until the set of eight to ten repetitions is complete. Take a deep breath, wait 15 to 30 seconds and begin your next set.

Common Errors

- Poor posture: shoulders rounded; head down
- Not having the chest against the pad
- Lifting too much weight
- Improper adjustment of the seat
- Not having entire upper arm on the pad
- Not pausing after each repetition when the elbow is extended
- Elbow hyperextended at the beginning of the repetition
- Not breathing during the exercise
- Not tightening abdominal muscles before lifting the weight
- Not performing the lift with full range of motion
- Performing the initial phase of the exercise too quickly
- Dropping the weight to the starting position too quickly instead of slowly controlling it
- Using the upper torso, instead of the biceps and upper arm, to perform the work

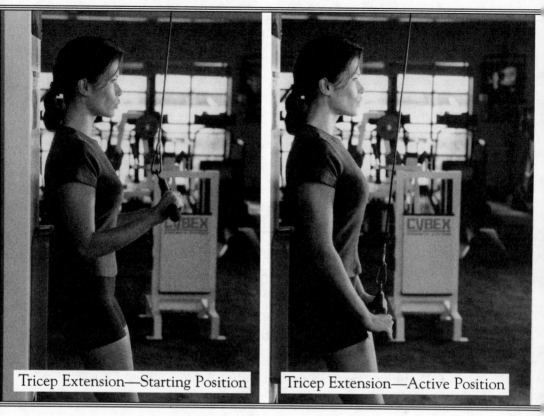

Tricep Extension—Starting Position | Tricep Extension—Active Position

Primary muscles involved:

Triceps

Starting position Stand erect against the back pad with your feet shoulder width apart. Knees should be slightly bent. Grasp the bar using an overhand grip with your hands three to five inches apart. The bar should be chest high and your elbows should be squeezing against your rib cage.

Active phase Contract your abdominal muscles before lifting the weight. While maintaining your posture, extend your forearms down until your wrists touch your thighs. Keep your elbows locked against your side. Return to the starting position gradually. Your wrists should remain straight throughout the exercise. Be sure to exhale while pressing the weight down and inhale on the return to the starting position. The initial lifting phase should take two to three seconds, as should the return to the starting position. When each repetition is complete, pause for a split second and start the next repetition. Continue until the set of eight to ten repetitions is complete. Take a deep breath, wait 15 to 30 seconds and begin your next set.

Common Errors

- Poor posture: shoulders rounded; head down; torso bent forward
- Not having the back flush against the pad
- Hands too far apart
- Bar moving too high above the chest
- Elbows moving away from the side
- Not pausing following each repetition when elbow is extended
- Elbows hyperextended at the beginning of the repetition
- Not breathing during the exercise
- Not tightening abdominal muscles before lifting the weight
- Not performing the lift with full range of motion
- Performing the initial phase of the exercise too quickly
- Returning the weight to the starting position too quickly instead of slowly controlling it
- Using the upper torso, instead of the triceps, to perform the work

Primary muscles involved:
Triceps and Shoulders

Starting position Adjust the seat so that the handles are level with your shoulders. Select your resistance. The body should be erect with the back firmly against the seat. Grasp the hand holds firmly. If there are two handle options, pick the one that allows your palms to face one another. This places less stress on your shoulders.

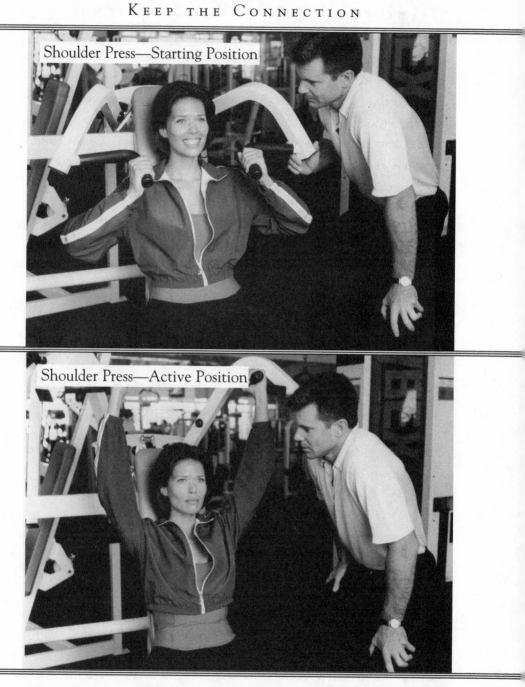

Shoulder Press—Starting Position

Shoulder Press—Active Position

Active phase Contract your abdominal muscles before lifting the weight. Push up to a complete extension. Your elbows should be directly under your wrists throughout the entire motion. Pause for a second at full extension, then return to the starting position gradually. Be sure to exhale on the extension phase, inhale on the return to the starting position. The extension phase should take two to three seconds, as should the return to the starting position. When each repetition is complete, pause for a split second and start the next repetition. Continue until the set of eight to ten repetitions is complete. Take a deep breath, wait 15 to 30 seconds and begin your next set.

Common Errors

- Poor posture: head down
- Allowing the back to lift off back pad
- Lifting too much weight
- Improper adjustment of the seat
- Arching the back while lifting
- Not breathing during the exercise
- Not tightening abdominal muscles before lifting the weight
- Not performing the lift with the full range of motion
- Performing the initial phase of the exercise too quickly
- Returning the weight to the starting position too quickly instead of slowly controlling it

Primary muscles involved:
Upper Back

Starting position Adjust the seat height so that the handle is at or slightly below shoulder height. Adjust the chest pad to allow the hands to grasp both handles and allow for the arms to be fully extended. Check the weight stack for the appropriate setting. Rest your chest against the pad. Grasp the lower end of the vertical handholds with palms facing in.

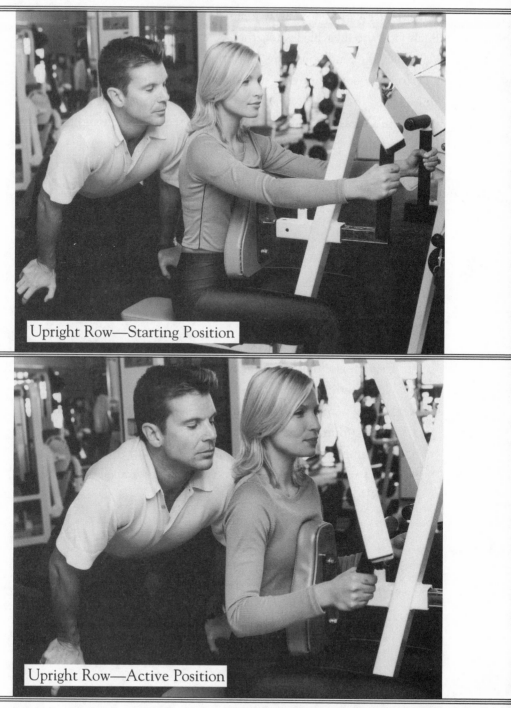

Upright Row—Starting Position

Upright Row—Active Position

Active phase Contract your abdominal muscles before lifting the weight. Pinch your shoulder blades together. Keep your chest pressed against the pad while you bend your arms and bring your elbows to the side of your body. Return your arms to the starting position gradually. Be sure to exhale while pulling toward you, inhale on the return to the starting position. The initial lifting phase should take two to three seconds, as should the return to the starting position. When each repetition is complete, pause for a split second and start the next repetition. Continue until the set of eight to ten repetitions is complete. Take a deep breath, wait 15 to 30 seconds and begin your next set.

Common Errors

- Poor posture: head down
- Not having the chest against the pad
- Lifting too much weight
- Improper seat adjustment
- Using torso to lift the weight
- Not breathing during the exercise
- Not tightening abdominal muscles before lifting the weight
- Not performing the lift with full range of motion
- Performing the initial phase of the exercise too quickly
- Returning the weight to the starting position too quickly instead of slowly controlling it

Name <u>Karen Miller</u>

Starting Date <u>June 1, 1999</u>

Body Weight <u>147</u>

Sample Workout Card (filled out)

RESISTANCE WORKOUT

	Exercise	Muscle Area	Sets	Set	Week # Day 1 1	2	3	Day 2 1	2	3	Day 3 1	2	3	Week # Day 1 1	2	3	Day 2 1	2	3	Day 3 1	2	3
1	Leg Press	Buttocks/ Quads/Ham	2	Wt.	90	90																
				Reps	10	8																
2	Leg Extension	Quads	2	Wt.	40	40																
				Reps	10	8																
3	Leg Curl	Hamstrings	2	Wt.	30	30																
				Reps	10	10																
4	Chest Press	Chest- Triceps	2	Wt.	35	35																
				Reps	10	10																
5	Bicep Curl	Biceps	2	Wt.	15	15																
				Reps	10	8																
6	Tricep Extension	Triceps	2	Wt.	10	10																
				Reps	10	8																
7	Shoulder Press	Shoulder/ Triceps	1	Wt.	30	30																
				Reps	10	10																
8	Upright Row	Upper Back	1	Wt.	40	40																
				Reps	10	8																
9	Basic Crunch	Abs	3	Wt.	N/A	N/A																
				Reps	15	15																
10	Twisting Trunk Curl	Abs	3	Wt.	N/A	N/A																
				Reps	15	15																
11				Wt.																		
				Reps																		
12				Wt.																		
				Reps																		

3. Nutrition

In our culture, we have become so driven by weight loss that we have forgotten about basic nutrition. We have made losing weight our focus, instead of doing what is best for our overall health. But when you do what is best for your health, you will naturally shed pounds and reach the best weight for you.

It's time that we made good health our priority. Let's think of nutrition as nourishment. When you nourish yourself, you are really nurturing yourself. You are attending to your body's needs. You are not only sustaining the body, but you are doing what is good for it.

Let's forget about dieting once and for all. People always ask me questions about a particular diet, usually whichever one is in vogue—and there have been a lot since *Make the Connection* was published. It seems a new "method" of eating comes along every few months. Most of them are old ideas repackaged to look new. Simply insert any fad food here, and you can name about half of them. Most of these diet plans prey on people who are desperate to lose weight, but they also attract people looking for a quick way to lose a few pounds. Sure, they all work—for a little while. But what does it cost you in the end—pain and aggravation because you're depriving yourself? Embarrassment and a slap to your self-esteem when you gain the weight back? Or worse, your health?

Just look at the popular high-protein, low-carbohydrate diets. With many of them, you can eat more meat and eggs than you ever thought you could. Besides the fact that in the long run these diets are hard on your body, especially your liver and kidneys, they usually have you eating an unhealthy amount of fat, increasing your risk for both heart disease and cancer. But at least you'll look better, right? Yes, you will probably lose weight on these plans, a lot of it from water and carbohydrates stored in your muscle. But the loss of both of these nutrients takes away from your health and your ability to exercise effectively. And I believe that exercise is essential to living a vibrant life.

Let me make it simple for you when deciding how to eat: Do what is best for your overall health. Not very revolutionary, huh? Most of us already know how to do that, yet we're still looking for miracles. We're looking in the wrong places. The answer is not outside ourselves. It's been inside of us the whole time. The answer to being healthy and fit lies in our desire and drive to change and better ourselves. The real miracle is when we put our minds to doing what is good and healthy for us and, in doing so, actually change our bodies and our lives.

It's really all about common sense. Come on, you didn't really think that any diet that tells you to limit the amount of fruits and vegetables you eat would be good for your overall health! We were meant to eat a variety of foods. Our bodies need so many nutrients—in combinations that we don't even know about yet—which is why it's so important to have a diverse diet. The key to healthy eating is to recognize that:

- We need variety
- There are virtually unlimited choices out there
- We can eat anything we wish, but our health, to a great degree, is affected by our choices

So, if you're concerned about your overall health and well-being, it is simply a matter of making wise choices—consistently. That's it. That is the key to nutrition. It sounds simple, but for many of us, actually living by those words is not an easy thing to do. We've picked up our bad eating habits over a period of years, so we can't expect them to change overnight. But changing them is what you must do if you want to make a lasting difference in your life.

Having said that, I don't want you to feel like you have to monitor everything you eat to the point that it takes all the joy out of eating. Nor should you feel as if going out to dinner or taking a vacation is impossible. That is what some diets do: They are temporary interruptions in your life. I'm asking you to simply make healthy choices most of the time. I'm not concerned with every little thing you eat, nor am I telling you that there are some things you can never eat. I'm concerned with the way you eat most of the time. If you stray every once in a while, fine. What's important is what you do consistently. It's the same with exercise: The results are in consistency.

I would guess that there are choices in everyone's diets that could be improved. The wonderful thing about nutrition is that it does not have to be perfect overnight. You can continually improve your diet by making better choices. Most of you have the knowledge you need to make good choices; just about all of us have heard of the basic food groups and know about getting fat out of our diets. Still, it can't hurt to be reminded. Remember, health is our number one concern. When it comes to eating, I want you to commit to the following sentence. Say it and live it:

I am going to eat a variety of healthy foods in reasonable portions.

That's all you need to do. But now, let's get a little more specific. In the ultimate healthy eating plan, you will want to incorporate these seven practices:

Eat only three meals and two snacks each day
Stop eating two to three hours before bedtime
Eat within the recommended guidelines from the food guide pyramid
Actively limit the amount of fat in your diet

Keep the Connection

Actively limit the amount of sugar in your diet

Drink eight glasses of water each day

Actively limit or eliminate the use of alcohol

These seven principles are building blocks to a healthy life. Adopt them and you will significantly improve your health and well-being. You may recognize most of these practices from *Make the Connection* as steps to effective weight loss. This is no coincidence. The simple truth is, by following these principles and exercising, you can reach any goal you have. And, whatever the goal, the best path to follow is always the one that puts your overall health first. Now, let's learn a little about each of the seven principles.

Eat only three meals and two snacks each day

Should I or should I not eat breakfast? I'm asked this question all the time, and the answer is always yes. When you eat three meals—breakfast, lunch and dinner—and two snacks, you are spreading your calories throughout the day. A lot of people think they have to deprive themselves of food in order to lose weight. That's wrong. If you withhold food from your body, it will work against you. That's because your metabolism needs food to keep it elevated. Deprive your metabolism, such as when you're on a low-calorie diet, and it responds by shutting down. Eating actually *raises* your metabolism.

You need to eat. It's best to eat smaller meals, more frequently. Some of you are in the habit of eating just one large meal a day. You're giving your metabolism one little boost, and for the rest of the day it is essentially shut down. Here's an example: You skip breakfast and lunch, omit all snacks, then eat a huge dinner. Your metabolism gears up at dinnertime, but that's all. What's worse, when you eat a large quantity of food at one sitting, your body produces even more insulin than usual, which takes the excess calories your body doesn't use and converts them into fat. You're defeating your own intentions.

Those of you who distribute your calories throughout the day are giving your metabolism a boost at each meal. So it works harder for you—all day. And you're not subject to the insulin "spike" you get by eating one large meal. If you spread your meals throughout the day, you do not send a signal to your body to deposit fat. But if you eat just one or a couple meals a day, you tell your body to store fat. The message is simple: Eat three meals and two snacks each day!

What about eating before your morning workout? If you're like me, you'll need a little snack before you exercise. This is not considered one of your two snacks; in essence, it's an optional third snack. It might be some fruit, an English muffin (or half), or perhaps some fruit juice. You should have it soon after you wake up, so that by the time you dress for your workout and stretch, you will be ready to exercise. Some people, however, simply can't tolerate eating first thing in the morning before exercising. It's an individual matter.

Let's go back to the breakfast question. As I said earlier, it's a good idea to distribute your calories throughout the day. It's also a good idea to eat more of those calories early in the day. Traditionally, we have a small breakfast, or skip it altogether; a somewhat larger lunch; and by far our largest meal at dinner. Then we make it worse by doing most of our power snacking late at night. This is a good way to pack on the most pounds. Also, food eaten late in the evening sits around undigested all night. Besides being gross, it's just plain unhealthy. We'll talk about that in more detail in a later section.

What we should all be doing is eating a solid breakfast, a solid lunch, two or three snacks and a smaller dinner. Our meals should consist of approximately the same amount of calories. And your snacks should be just that; they shouldn't look like fourth and fifth meals. I've included some snack suggestions in the "Recipes" section.

Stop eating two to three hours before bedtime

Your body's metabolism changes slightly throughout the day. In the morning, it is relatively slow. As your day goes on, your metabolism increases, until it peaks in the evening. When you sleep, your metabolism decreases to its slowest level, until just before you wake up. Then the entire cycle starts all over again.

Both eating and exercising boost your metabolism. I recommend that you exercise in the morning, in part because it gets your metabolism going early and you burn a higher rate of calories all day long. For the same reason, I suggest moving more of your calories toward breakfast and lunch and away from dinner. Again, it will rev up your metabolism early in the day.

So why not add calories at dinner and bedtime to further boost your metabolism? It appears that your metabolism does not increase to the same extent in response to eating late in the day. In theory, calories eaten late in the day are just waiting around to be converted to fat. It's almost as if your body knows that sleep is inevitable and it does not want to be "revved up." And, once you do fall asleep, your metabolism plummets, regardless of what you've eaten. Why this happens is not yet fully understood. But the belief is that your body reaches a metabolic maximum late in the day—perhaps to prepare for impending sleep. So calories eaten late in the day or, worse, around bedtime will be converted to fat more quickly. Furthermore, when food remains in your stomach and intestines for too long, it increases your risk for various cancers.

I have noticed through the years that clients who are able to stop eating two to three hours before bedtime are much more successful at losing weight and keeping it off than those who eat later at night and at bedtime. With almost all of these clients, it was a challenge at first to eliminate late-night eating.

I saw it with myself. Even though I have been very active all my life, when I first started eliminating my late-evening eating, I immediately dropped three pounds. That's a lot for me! Those three pounds never come back unless I start eating within two hours of bedtime.

There's no doubt: It's in your best interest to adopt this principle. A technique some people use to successfully combat late night cravings is to distract themselves with something satisfying—other than food. It might be drinking a cup of herbal tea or taking a hot bubble bath. Another great technique is to visualize yourself getting thinner or healthier because you are resisting these cravings. Before you know it, your visualization will become a reality.

All of this may require you to change your current habits, but that's what we're talking about. Experiment with different times regarding your meals and snacks. Eventually you will come up with the perfect system for you. Just remember, do not eat two to three hours before bedtime! You will not only improve your health, but you'll feel better and sleep better, too.

Eat within the recommended guidelines from the Food Guide Pyramid

Whether we are eating at home or dining out, we Americans eat way too much. Yet we limit the kinds of food we eat. We've grown accustomed to consuming large quantities from a narrow range of choices. It's true. We are growing as a nation, not only in numbers but in body size. Did you know that chairs are being made larger? I'm talking about chairs we buy for our homes, airline seats, even stadium bleachers. Obviously, this is due to the fact that we're eating more and we're eating more often. We're also exercising less. Studies show that people who eat less, relative to their activity level, live longer and healthier lives. Isn't that what we all want? If so, it's in our best interest to control our eating. Having said that, I want you to know that there is a wide selection of foods you can choose from. All you have to do is open your mind and follow these guidelines:

The Food Guide Pyramid—The guidelines I like best are outlined in the Food Guide Pyramid, developed by the United States Department of Agriculture. It's an easy-to-follow plan that lists the types and amounts of foods you should consume daily. There are six basic food categories, along with recommended servings for each category (except the Fats, Oils and Sweets Group). Some of you may already be familiar with the pyramid, but I find it to be the simplest, most flexible way to present this information. And once you learn it, it becomes a natural way to eat—just as eating should be! The pyramid is shown below:

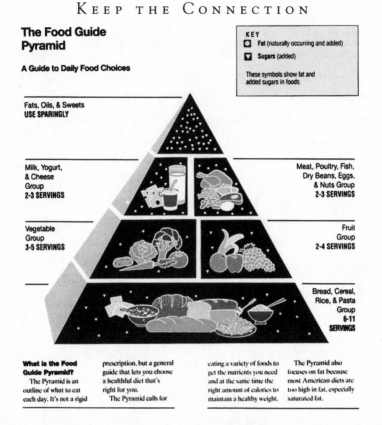

The Food Guide Pyramid

A Guide to Daily Food Choices

KEY
☐ Fat (naturally occurring and added)
▼ Sugars (added)

These symbols show fat and added sugars in foods.

Fats, Oils, & Sweets
USE SPARINGLY

Milk, Yogurt, & Cheese Group
2-3 SERVINGS

Meat, Poultry, Fish, Dry Beans, Eggs, & Nuts Group
2-3 SERVINGS

Vegetable Group
3-5 SERVINGS

Fruit Group
2-4 SERVINGS

Bread, Cereal, Rice, & Pasta Group
6-11 SERVINGS

What is the Food Guide Pyramid?
The Pyramid is an outline of what to eat each day. It's not a rigid prescription, but a general guide that lets you choose a healthful diet that's right for you.

The Pyramid calls for eating a variety of foods to get the nutrients you need and at the same time the right amount of calories to maintain a healthy weight.

The Pyramid also focuses on fat because most American diets are too high in fat, especially saturated fat.

To use the pyramid, you need to eat within the guidelines of each food group. Keep in mind that the pyramid is just a guide. It may take some trial and error before you find the number of servings, within each group, that is right for you and suitable to your goals. Each day you should have between:

6–11 servings from the Bread, Cereal, Rice & Pasta Group
2–4 servings from the Fruit Group
3–5 servings from the Vegetable Group
2–3 servings from the Meat, Poultry, Fish, Dry Beans, Eggs & Nuts Group
2-3 servings from the Milk, Yogurt & Cheese Group
"Use sparingly" choices from the Fats, Oils & Sweets Group (Refer to the sections on eliminating fat and sugar)

Breads, Cereal, Rice & Pasta Group (6–11 servings) Sometimes I refer
to this group as the whole grains group, even though products made with
refined flour are included here. The best choices in this group are always
products derived from whole grains, such as whole grain breads and cereals.
More of their nutritional value is intact, and they contain more fiber.

One serving equals:

> 1 slice of bread
> ½ cup of cooked cereal, rice or pasta
> 1 oz. of breakfast cereal
> 1 oz. of pretzels (about one large Bavarian pretzel)

Fruit Group (2–4 servings) This group includes all fresh fruit as well as
canned and dried fruit and fruit juice. Fresh fruit is the best choice since it
is loaded with vitamins, minerals, water and fiber. Fruit juice is also a good
choice. I prefer citrus such as orange and grapefruit juice, and the more
pulp, the better. Canned fruit should be eaten infrequently or not at all,
since it is usually packed in sugar. Dried fruits are okay as a snack, but
should be eaten only occasionally, since they have less nutrients, and take
up less space in your stomach than fresh fruits, potentially causing you to
eat more of them.

One serving equals:

> 1 cup strawberries, raspberries, blackberries, boysenberries
> 1 medium-size apple, orange, pear, peach, grapefruit, or apricot
> 1 6-oz. glass of fruit juice
> 1 cup cooked or canned fruit
> 1 banana
> 1 cup grapes

Vegetable Group (3–5 servings) This group includes all fresh, frozen and canned vegetables. Fresh vegetables are always preferred to frozen and canned since they are higher in vitamins, minerals, water and fiber. Frozen is acceptable and a better choice than canned. Make it a point to limit or eliminate the use of canned vegetables.

Like many of you, I grew up eating some canned vegetables. As a kid, I didn't much like vegetables, but I especially detested the canned variety. One time, when I was about 11, I sneaked into the kitchen cabinet and switched all the labels on the canned vegetables. I carefully removed each of the labels, then meticulously pasted them on different cans. My mother discovered my little prank when she opened a can of beets and found creamed corn instead. I no longer have to go to such lengths to avoid canned vegetables. Now I only eat them fresh. Not only do they taste better, but they are healthier for you too.

One serving equals:

> ½ cup raw or cooked broccoli, corn, Brussels sprouts,
> green beans or squash
> 6 oz. or ¾ cup tomato or carrot juice
> Lettuce, tomato and onion (on a sandwich)
> 1 cup leafy vegetables (as a base for a salad)

Meat, Poultry, Fish, Dry Beans, Eggs & Nuts Group (2–4 servings) I like to refer to this group as the high-quality protein group. Even though this group includes choices that can be high in fat and low in protein, you should select choices that are high in protein, low in fat. These include skinless chicken and turkey, lean cuts of beef and, occasionally, pork. As for eggs, you should eat the egg white, as opposed to the entire egg. Eggs are one of the best sources of protein. You can get most of the benefits of them in the egg white, without the additional cholesterol in the yolk. Nuts are also part of this group, but they should be eaten on an infrequent basis because they are high in fat and, typically, salt.

One serving equals:

    3 oz. beef, chicken or pork
    1 cup cooked beans (black beans, black-eyed peas, red beans, etc.)
    3 oz. cooked fish
    3 eggs (whites only)

Milk, Yogurt & Cheese Group (2–3 servings) This is a group in which you can trim away a lot of fat! You should have skim or 1 percent milk instead of 2 percent or whole milk. Soy milk, which has become more readily available, is also a great choice. Recent studies suggest that soy products may decrease your risk for various cancers, particularly breast cancer. Other good selections from this group include low fat yogurt, cheese or cottage cheese. And for dessert, choose frozen yogurt or sorbet over ice cream.

One serving equals:

    8 oz. milk
    8 oz. yogurt
    1 oz. cheese (natural cheese; 2 oz. processed cheese)
    ½ cup cottage cheese

Fats, Oils & Sweets Group This group includes canola oil, olive oil, palm oil, lard—any fat that you can cook with. It also includes sweets such as cakes, pies, candy, pastries and, in general, foods high in sugar content. You will notice that this group does not have a number of recommended servings. That's because the less you eat from this group, the better. I'll discuss how to limit fat and sugar in your diet in later sections. Since all the fat you need is typically provided for by eating within the ranges of the other groups, the ideal number of servings from this group would be zero. For some people, achieving that may be difficult at first. If this is the case for you, gradually reduce the number of servings from this group until you reach the lowest amount you are willing to consume. Limiting servings from this group is one of the best things you can do for your weight-loss program and your health—which is why I will discuss it in more detail soon.

The food pyramid is an excellent guide to what makes a nutritious, well-balanced diet for most people. I am going to suggest a couple of tips that can work well right alongside the food pyramid.

- Milk should be skim, 1 percent or soy.
- Yogurt and cheese should be low fat.
- Meats should be lean cuts with the excess fat trimmed off.
- Nuts should be avoided.
- Eat up to six vegetables a day.
- Two or even three servings of fruit is best.
- Limit the servings of bread to one per meal.
- Limit your bread, cereal, rice and pasta to six to eight servings per day.

A Healthy Eating Day:

Breakfast
　　1 oz. cereal mix with approximately ½ cup of skim, 1 percent or soy milk
　　8 oz. glass of orange juice
　　Herbal tea

Lunch
　　Red Pepper with Grilled Corn Soup
　　Barbecue Chicken Sandwich
　　8 oz. glass of skim or 1 percent milk

Snack
　　1 oz. pretzels or 1 Bavarian pretzel (with salsa or mustard)

Dinner

    Eggplant with Chicken

    1 cup broccoli (counts as 2 servings)

    1 cup couscous

    Slice of sourdough bread

    8 oz. glass of water with lemon wedge

Snack

    1 cup mixed berries (strawberries, blueberries, boysenberries)

Total servings

    Bread, cereal, rice, pasta group 6

    Fruit group 2

    Vegetable group 5

    Milk, Yogurt & Cheese group 2

    Meat, Poultry, Fish, Dry Beans, Eggs & Nuts group 2

The recipes for this healthy eating day are included in the back of the book.

Actively limit the amount of fat in your diet

For those of you concerned about counting fat grams and eating low fat foods, understand that we actually need some fat in our diet. Fat assists in our digestion, increases our immunity to disease, transports cholesterol and makes hormones. The problem comes when we get too much fat in our diets. Fat is a high-calorie nutrient. It contains more than double the amount of calories that you find in equal amounts of carbohydrates or protein.

Getting most of the fat out of your diet is essential for improving your overall health. High-fat diets contribute not only to our weight, but to the risk of cancer and heart disease. We should all strive to reduce the amount of total fat consumed in a day to between 20 and 50 grams.

All or most of the fat you eat should come from unsaturated sources such as olive oil, safflower oil, canola oil—oil from plant sources. The tropical oils—coconut and palm oil—are also from plant sources, but should be avoided since they are saturated. Other saturated fat sources—butter, lard and the fat found on animal meat—should be limited or eliminated from your diet.

You really have a relatively wide range to work with here. If you consume 50 grams of fat, you are consuming two and a half times as much fat as someone who is eating 20 grams of fat. But since we all have different energy needs and different genetic makeups, what works for one person may not necessarily work for another. This has been the downfall of many eating or weight-loss systems. They try to tell us what works for everyone. As a side note, 50 grams of fat per day is higher than I would like to see anyone consume on an ongoing basis, but represents a reasonable first goal for many people.

You can even reduce your fat intake by too much. If, for example, you constantly crave foods that are high in fat, never feel satisfied with your meals or your skin becomes very dry, you may need to increase the amount of fat in your diet. Be sure to give yourself some time to adjust, however, because whenever you cut down on anything, your body misses it for a while. Our bodies give us constant feedback. We just need to learn how to listen to them.

Start by reducing your fat intake to about 50 grams a day—unless you already consume less. For some of you this may mean a significant reduction in your total fat intake. If so, it may be difficult cutting back at first. I have known people who routinely consume more than 200 fat grams a day. That's the same amount you would get if you ate about 2 ½ sticks of butter. If you are consuming more than 200 grams a day, any reduction in the amount of fat you eat is a positive step for your health. So, just gradually begin reducing your fat grams.

When you first start cutting back, you will probably find that you crave fat for a while. Again, that's because you are depriving your body of something it is used to having. These cravings will eventually go away. It takes a little time, but once you become more active and your body grows accustomed to having less fat, you won't even miss it. Just be patient!

Tracking the fat in your diet—While I don't believe you should count anything every day, when you are learning about what to eat and how much, it is helpful to count fat grams for a while. After about three months, most people no longer need to keep count. They automatically and quite naturally keep their fat consumption within the desired range.

In the meantime, you should have no problem keeping track of the amount of fat you eat. Food manufacturers have flooded the market with new, low fat items. And, as you are probably aware, all packaged foods have labels that contain nutritional information. The fat content will be expressed either in "calories from fat" or "grams of fat," or both. In one gram of fat there are nine calories. So, to convert calories from fat to grams of fat, simply divide the total calories from fat by nine. That will give you the amount of fat grams. It's also a good idea to have a fat gram chart, which lists hundreds of commonly eaten foods. You can find it at your local bookstore or health food store.

How much fat is right for you?—You should decide, within the guidelines, how much fat to take out of your diet. I suggest starting at the higher end of the range (35 to 50 grams a day), unless you are currently eating less. If you are already consuming below 50 grams, then start cutting back in increments of five grams. This should be done at your own pace. If you reduce your fat intake slowly, you give your body more time to adjust.

In general, the less fat you consume, the healthier your diet. But, for most people, going below 20 grams a day provides little benefit and can actually cause health problems. Your ultimate goal should be to keep your fat intake between 20 and 35 grams each day, with the majority of those grams coming from unsaturated sources. (If you are a pregnant or lactating woman, you should consult your physician for recommended fat intake.)

This is an ongoing process and could take one or even two years to accomplish. That's okay.

You might find it helpful to keep track of your fat intake using a journal. You can record what works and what doesn't, as well as how your body is responding to changes in both eating and exercise. Some of you may want to keep an even more accurate record of fat grams by basing your fat intake on the number of calories you are consuming. For you, I recommend that 10 to 20 percent of your total calories come primarily from unsaturated fat.

One last point about eating low fat: Don't be fooled into thinking the low fat label gives you permission to eat more. With all the new low fat products available, nutrition experts are concerned that people are eating more than they ordinarily would. If you do so, you may be consuming the same or even more total calories—defeating the purpose of eating low fat. Moreover, many foods packaged with less fat have higher amounts of sugar. Too much sugar can also be a health hazard. So be reasonable when it comes to eating low fat foods.

Actively limit the amount of sugar in your diet

The average American consumes well in excess of 100 pounds of refined sugar each year. Yes, you read that correctly: 100 pounds! Consuming too much sugar has been shown to:

- Cause weight gain and contribute to obesity
- Increase the incidence of diabetes
- Contribute to the progression of cardiovascular disease
- Contribute to the incidence of various cancers

And that's just what we know now! There is no question that limiting your consumption of sugar is in your best interest. We're going to look at some ways to do that, but first, let's talk about what sugar is.

Sugar is really carbohydrate. For some, this causes a good bit of confusion, since we've been told carbohydrates are good for us. The truth is, there are some carbohydrates that are bad for us and others that we need in our diet. To make sense of this, you might find it useful to learn a little about carbohydrates.

There are basically three different types of carbohydrates: monosaccharides, oligosaccharides and polysaccharides. They are distinguished by the number of simple sugars that they are made of.

Monosaccharides are simple sugars: glucose, fructose and galactose. Glucose, also known as blood sugar, can be produced when your body breaks down more complex carbohydrates. It's also found in some of the foods we eat.

Oligosaccharides are most frequently disaccharides or double sugars. They are formed when two monosaccharides combine. The three main disaccharides are:

Lactose = glucose + galactose

Maltose = glucose + glucose

Sucrose = glucose + fructose

Lactose is the sugar found in milk. It's also referred to as milk sugar. Maltose is not a common component to our diets. It shows up in malt products, such as beer and certain germinating cereals. Sucrose is the most common dietary sugar and is abundant in cane sugar, honey, brown sugar, maple syrup, even beets. We should be most concerned about limiting sucrose in our diet—and be particularly aware of limiting refined sugar or table sugar. Refined sugar comes from stripping the natural coating from the cane plant and is found abundantly in foods such as candy, cakes, pies, soda and some cereals.

Polysaccharides occur when three or more simple sugars are combined and can be made up of hundreds of simple sugars connected to each other. They are found in both plants and animals. In animals, polysaccharides are made and stored in the muscles for energy. We call this animal carbohydrate glycogen.

When we speak of complex carbohydrates, we are typically referring to plant polysaccharides. In plants, there are two types of polysaccharides: cellulose and starch. Cellulose is the fibrous part of the plant. We know it as fiber. It's good to get plenty of fiber in your diet. You can get it from sources such as leafy vegetables, pulp and the skin on most fruits.

Starch is abundant in our diets. It's found in such foods as potatoes, corn, bread, cereal, beans, peas, rice and pasta. Some people feel they should avoid starch, when, in fact, this complex carbohydrate is very important to our diet and our health. I suggest that about 50 percent of your total calories come from complex carbohydrates as opposed to simple sugars. Unfortunately, there's been an unhealthy trend toward decreasing complex carbohydrates in favor of simple sugars. **Your goal should be to limit your intake of simple sugars—sucrose, in particular—while increasing your consumption of complex carbohydrates.**

Be aware, though, that just as there is refined sugar, there are processed grain products, such as white rice, white flour and white bread. They are much lower in nutritional value than whole grains, and should be avoided. Whole grain breads, brown or whole grain rice and whole grain pastas are much better choices.

I don't believe it's necessary to keep a record of your sugar intake in the same way you would keep track of your fat grams. Most people do fine if they just know what to avoid.

Avoid
   Table (refined) sugar
   Soda
   Candy
   Cake
   Pie
   White flour
   Processed grain products, such as:
    Pastas
    White rice
    White bread

Healthy choices

Fruits

Vegetables

Beans/legumes

Whole grain breads

Whole grain pastas

Whole grain rice

Brown rice

Drink eight glasses of water each day

Water is the body's most important nutrient. It is literally essential to life. Without it, we would survive maybe two to three days. Ideally, water should make up about 60 percent of your body weight. Because we lose so much of it just through basic body functions—and even more through exercise—it is important to replenish the supply by drinking more water. That is why I recommend drinking eight glasses of water a day. When your body's water supply cannot meet its demands, you become dehydrated, which can cause a variety of complications, including heat exhaustion and heatstroke.

Water is also essential to many of the body's functions. It's particularly important in controlling your weight because it both improves digestion and helps metabolize fat. Water also fills you up. Drinking eight glasses will help curb your appetite so that you don't overeat. Also, there are times when you are dehydrated and your body may signal you to eat, when what it really requires is water. I call this phenomenon artificial hunger. By meeting all of your nutritional needs, including your need for water, you can control artificial hunger.

You can also exercise more effectively and at higher levels when you are getting enough water. In fact, water becomes more important the more active you are. For one thing, as you gain muscle, which is comprised of about 70 percent water, you will require more water and need to replace more of it daily. Think of it as a cycle: The more muscle you maintain, the more water is held by the body and the more water you must consume. Within those muscles is the carbohydrate glycogen, which also increases as you become more fit. Every gram of glycogen holds about 2.5 to 3 grams of water. The bottom line is, the more fit you are, the more water your body will hold, and the more water you need each day.

Unfortunately, our bodies' thirst mechanism does not always tell us when we are thirsty. By the time we experience thirst, our bodies are already in a slight state of dehydration. And even after our thirst is satisfied, we may still be somewhat dehydrated. You should drink your eight glasses in moderate-sized portions (8-ounce glasses) throughout the course of the day, instead of drinking them all at once. When you drink large quantities of water at one time, you stimulate the body to rid itself of water.

We get water from three primary sources: liquids (water, of course; juice, milk, soda, etc.); almost all the foods we eat (fruits and vegetables contain the most); and our metabolism, when it breaks down a source of energy (producing carbon dioxide and water). But I still want you to drink eight (8-ounce) glasses of fresh, noncarbonated water a day. True, water is found in other beverages, but these should be in addition to your eight glasses. Also, try to limit the amount of caffeinated beverages you consume, since caffeine is a strong diuretic and stimulates your body to release water. Try herbal tea instead of regular tea or coffee. There was a time I considered carbonated (sparkling) water an acceptable source for water, but because of its diuretic effect, you really shouldn't count it toward your eight glasses a day.

Follow these simple guidelines and you can be sure of getting enough water. And don't worry about getting too much water; your body will get rid of the excess. Drinking eight glasses a day becomes easier the more active you are.

Here's a perfect water day:

Start with a glass of water before your workout. You'll probably be thirsty after your workout, so have two more glasses. Have two between breakfast and lunch and you're already over halfway toward your daily goal. Have another glass during lunch and another one between lunch and dinner. Then finish off your day with a glass at dinner. This makes a total of eight glasses. If you prefer to sip water all day, carry it with you in a bottle. Just make sure you drink your eight glasses!

Actively limit or eliminate the use of alcohol

You may already be thinking I'm a stair-stepping, weight-pumping, sprout-eating fitness fanatic. And, to top it off, you're thinking, I'm a teetotaler too. Well, the first part is somewhat accurate. I like using the stairs, and I put in my time in the weight room, and I've eaten a sprout or two and, yes, I like talking about fitness. But I also enjoy the occasional glass of wine.

When I do indulge, I'm fully aware of its effects on my body. Let's face it, alcohol has some strikes against it when it comes to your health and fitness. First, alcohol is quite high in calories—it's only slightly better than pure fat. This is illustrated below for you:

Carbohydrates = 4 calories per gram

Protein = 4 calories per gram

Alcohol = 7 calories per gram

Fat = 9 calories per gram

The second strike against alcohol is, it doesn't fill you up. It's absorbed from the stomach into the bloodstream almost immediately. So instead, you fill up on food, further increasing the total calories you consume.

Worst of all, alcohol slows your metabolism. After all, it's a depressant. In fact, the effects of drinking alcohol can actually linger for days after overindulging, which could mean you're not going to feel much like working out. You will be much more willing, and likely, to abandon your program of healthy living—at least until the alcohol wears off.

For all of those reasons, the best recommendation is to eliminate alcohol altogether. If you are not willing to eliminate it entirely, then at least cut your consumption in half. Simply estimate what you drink weekly and divide it by two. Really, it's the first drink that tastes the best. If you stop to think about it, you'll see the subsequent drinks are not worth the damage.

Some of you may have heard that one or two glasses of wine a day is actually good for your health, particularly your heart. You also may have heard that a couple glasses of wine a day can lower your cholesterol. This is still being debated. In fact, there are studies supporting both sides of the argument. One thing you should know is that a lot of these studies are taking into account a more sedentary population who are at higher risk for heart and cholesterol problems. In my opinion, a program of eating right and exercising would have a much greater positive effect on their health. But, even if alcohol is beneficial for certain people, we shouldn't take this as a license to overindulge. What is certain is that too much alcohol is bad on your heart, liver and other parts of the body. I also find that, in general, when you limit or eliminate alcohol from your life, you show a net increase in your overall health.

So, to help you cut back, consider using less alcohol in your drinks, such as making a wine spritzer with sparkling water. Or try alternative products, such as non-alcoholic beer or a club soda with lime, when you're at a party. Also, if you eat a meal before attending a social event, you will feel less like drinking.

When you do begin to cut back, you will be even less willing to imbibe, since you'll feel alcohol's ill effects to an even greater extent. And the fitter you become, the more sensitive you are to alcohol—kind of like putting cheap gas in your high-performance car. Remember, the more you restrict your alcohol consumption, the better your overall health will be.

4. Recipes

Making a healthy, well-balanced meal doesn't have to be difficult. I have put together some delicious menu ideas with recipes that are simple and easy to make. Enjoy! Please note that each recipe includes nutritional information such as calories, grams of fat, grams of protein and grams of carbohydrates. These estimated averages are based per serving and may differ slightly from product to product and from varying sizes of fresh ingredients.

Breakfast

MENU 1
Healthy Cereal Mix
Fresh blueberries
Soy, skim or 1 percent milk
Glass of orange juice (6–8 oz.)

MENU 2
Oatmeal
Strawberries or 1 banana
Glass of grapefruit juice (6–8 oz.)

MENU 3
Fruit Smoothie
Cup of herbal tea

MENU 4
Egg-White Omelet
Whole wheat toast
Healthy potatoes
Glass of orange juice (6–8 oz.)

Healthy Cereal Mix

With the busy lives most of us lead, we often need quick, easy-to-prepare break-fasts that are nutritious and taste good. The Healthy Cereal Mix fits the bill. I have selected all of the following cereals based on their nutritional value and the fact that there is no added sugar. The cereal mix is a great way to start your day with virtually no preparation time.

> ¼ cup Post Spoon-Size Shredded Wheat cereal
> ¼ cup Post Grape-Nuts cereal
> ¼ cup Quaker Puffed Rice cereal

Combine the cereals listed above (for ¾ cup total) in a bowl. Add approximately ½ cup of skim, 1 percent or soy milk and enjoy!

Some other cereals that you can substitute for the ones listed above are: Kellog's Nutri-Grain Golden Wheat cereal, General Mills Fiber One, Post Shredded Wheat and Bran, Post Grape-Nuts Flakes and Quaker Puffed Wheat.

(Note that 1 serving of cereal = ¾ cup: mix any number of cereals from the above list to make your ¾-cup serving.)

TIPS: The best way to make this cereal mix easy and convenient is to combine your favorite three cereals in a large plastic container with a tight fitting lid. Then it's always ready for you any time.

SOME CEREAL NUTRITION INFORMATION (FOR ¼ CUP)
Kellogg's Nutri-Grain Golden Wheat: Calories 45, Fat .15 g, Protein 1.5g, Carbohydrate 12g
Post Spoon-Size Shredded Wheat: Calories 23, Fat .15g, Protein .7g, Carbohydrate 5.6g

RECIPES

Post Grape-Nuts: Calories: 105, Fat .1g, Protein 3.1g, Carbohydrate .1g
Quaker Puffed Rice: Calories: 13, Fat .025g, Protein .25g, Carbohydrate 3.1g

PREP TIME: *5 minutes*
YIELD: *1 serving*
NUTRITION TOTALS: *Calories 141, Fat .275g, Protein 4.05g,*
Carbohydrate 31.8g

Oatmeal

This breakfast staple is a nutritious, hearty way to begin your day. Depending on your taste preference and the amount of time you have, you can select instant oatmeal, done in about 30 seconds; the original Quaker Oats–type, which takes about ten minutes; and natural grain oatmeal such as McCann's Irish Oatmeal, which can take about 30 minutes. As you probably guessed, my favorite is the natural grain oatmeal for its nutritional value as well as taste.

> 4 cups water
> 1 cup oatmeal (Irish or natural grain)
> 1 cinnamon stick
> ½ banana or ½ cup of fresh strawberries or your favorite fresh fruit

In a medium-size saucepan, bring water to a rapid boil. Stir in oatmeal and cinnamon stick. Reduce heat and simmer for about 30 minutes, or according to package directions, stirring often. Oatmeal is ready when it is creamy and smooth. Remove cinnamon stick before serving. Substituting skim or 1 percent milk for water makes a richer oatmeal. Vanilla soy milk, in particular, adds a unique flavor to this hot cereal. Be sure to add bananas, strawberries or any of your favorite fruits to the dish.

TIPS: Soak natural grain oatmeal overnight. It cuts the cooking time in half. If you like your oatmeal thicker, use less water. Overcooking weakens the nutty flavor of oatmeal.

PREP TIME: *Varies according to type of oatmeal. See breakdown.*
YIELD: *See breakdown*

Quaker Instant Oatmeal
PREP TIME: *1 minute*
YIELD: *1 ½ cups*

RECIPES

MAKES 1 SERVING

NUTRITION TOTALS: *Calories 100, Fat 2g, Protein 4g, Carbohydrate 19g*

Quaker Old-Fashioned Oats

PREP TIME: *5 to 10 minutes*

YIELD: *1 ½ cups*

MAKES 1 SERVING

NUTRITION TOTALS: *Calories 150, Fat 3g, Protein 5g, Carbohydrate 27g*

McCann's Irish Oatmeal

PREP TIME: *30 minutes*

YIELD: *3 cups*

MAKES 2 TO 3 SERVINGS

NUTRITION TOTALS: *Calories 145, Fat 2.4g, Protein 6g, Carbohydrate 25.2g*

Fruit Smoothie

In keeping with the idea that breakfast needs to be eaten each day and that time in the morning is at a premium, one of my favorite morning meals is a fruit smoothie. It provides for a quick, complete, nutritious breakfast.

½ medium papaya, peeled and seeded
1 medium ripe banana
1 cup fresh strawberries, stems removed
½ cup low or nonfat yogurt
½ orange, deseeded and juiced, or ½ cup orange juice
¾ cup ice cubes

Options:
¼ cup protein powder
¼ cup chopped nuts

In a blender or food processor, blend papaya, banana, strawberries, yogurt and orange juice for about 1 minute or until the mixture is smooth. Add any options, if desired, and blend for another minute. Add the ice and pulse until smooth and creamy. Serve in a chilled glass.

PREP TIME: *8 minutes*
YIELD: *2 ½ cups*
MAKES 2 SERVINGS
NUTRITION TOTALS: *Calories 164, Fat 1.8g, Protein 5.1g, Carbohydrate 35g*

Egg-White Omelet

The egg-white omelet may take a little more time to prepare than the previously featured breakfast items, but it represents a nutritious way to start your day. And it can be custom-designed to incorporate your favorite healthy fillings.

> Nonfat oil spray
> 2 teaspoons diced onions
> 1 medium mushroom, diced
> ½ tomato, diced
> Pinch freshly ground black pepper
> 8 egg whites, beaten

Options:
> ½ cup low fat cheese
> ½ cup Shiitake mushrooms, diced
> ½ cup portobello mushrooms, diced

In a medium-size pan sprayed with oil (avoid corn oil, which turns the egg whites yellowish), briefly sauté onions and mushroom over medium-high heat. Add tomatoes and black pepper and continue sautéing until most of the liquid cooks off. Set aside. Spray a 10-inch omelet pan with oil and warm it over medium heat for about 1 minute. Add egg whites and stir, occasionally tipping the pan to spread the eggs evenly until the mixture begins to firm up. Spread on filling, including low-fat cheese, if desired, and cook until the eggs are firm. Run a spatula along the sides and bottom of the omelet to loosen it from the pan. Remove the pan from the heat, tilt it sideways to position half the omelet onto a plate, then flip the pan upside down to roll the rest of the omelet into a half moon.

TIPS: Egg Beaters can be used as a substitute for egg whites. An egg-white omelet also is great at lunch or dinner.

RECIPES

PREP TIME: *20 minutes*

YIELD: *4 cups*

MAKES 2 SERVINGS

NUTRITION TOTALS: *Calories 80, Fat .2g, Protein 18g, Carbohydrate 2.5*

Breakfast Potatoes

As a perfect accompaniment to your omelet, breakfast potatoes are a hearty way to begin your morning.

1 pound new potatoes
nonfat oil spray
2 medium shallots, diced
½ medium green pepper, diced
½ medium red pepper, diced
1 teaspoon Cajun spice
Options:
1 strip turkey bacon
6 asparagus spears, trimmed and cut into 1-inch pieces

In a large pot of water, bring potatoes to a boil. Cook over medium heat for about 10 minutes until easily pierced with a knife. Drain the potatoes and set aside. Cut cooled potatoes into bite-size chunks. In a large skillet sprayed with oil, sauté shallots, peppers and spice for about 2 minutes. Stir in potatoes and cook until golden brown and crispy.

Adding 1 strip of turkey bacon to the boiling water adds a rich smoky character; it may also be diced and sautéed with potatoes. Asparagus adds a fresh green dimension to the medley.

PREP TIME: *40 minutes*
YIELD: *8 cups*
MAKES 4 SERVINGS
NUTRITION TOTALS: *Calories 56, Fat .7g, Protein 2.05g, Carbohydrate 9.35g*

Lunch

MENU 1

Red Pepper with Grilled Corn Soup

Smoked Turkey Sandwich

Herbal iced tea (8 oz.)

MENU 2

Vegetarian Pita Pocket

Potato-Spinach Soup

Glass of tomato juice (6–8 oz.)

MENU 3

Cold Crisp Penne Salad

Tomato-Basil Soup

Glass of cold apple cider (8 oz.)

Red Pepper with Grilled Corn Soup

If it were up to me, soup would be its own food group—I love it! And my all-time favorite soup is this one. I will say that this one does take a little extra effort but the result is well worth it.

Nonfat oil spray
5 medium red bell peppers, cored, seeded and coarsely chopped
1 medium onion, chopped
4 medium tomatoes, chopped
4 cups water or homemade chicken stock
4 tablespoons powdered chicken stock
2 ears fresh corn, husk removed, grilled and cut from cob
Salt and freshly ground pepper to taste
¼ teaspoon cayenne pepper

Options:
Roasted red peppers

In a large pot generously sprayed with oil, sauté the peppers and onion over medium-low heat for 8 minutes until limp but not browned (if using roasted peppers, scrape off crisped skin and deseed as usual). Stir in the tomatoes, cook another two minutes, and then add the water or homemade chicken stock. Simmer the mixture for about 20 minutes on low heat, occasionally skimming foam from the top. Stir in powdered stock and thoroughly blend it in (eliminate the soup powder if using homemade broth). Remove pot from heat and set aside.

Meanwhile, lightly spray the corn ears with oil, sprinkle them lightly with salt and pepper, and grill for about 8 minutes, turning constantly. Grilling may also be done on a cookie sheet in a 400 °F oven for about five minutes. In either method, the corn should be almost golden brown with a slight toasted aroma. With a sharp knife, trim off the kernels from the cooled corn and set them aside. (Peppers, too, may be roasted on a hot charcoal grill or directly on a cooking element. The crisp, blackened skin must be scraped off and seeds removed. This method imparts a smoky undertone to the flavor.)

While the corn is cooling, remove the pepper, onion and tomato mixture from the pot, and pulse it in a food processor or blender until smooth. (Do this in two batches to avoid overflow.) Retain the cooking liquid in the pot. With a fine-mesh sieve and the back of a spoon, re-strain the pulsed mixture to extract a fine pulp into the soup broth and discard the leftovers—mainly tough skin and tomato seeds.)

Return the soup pot to medium heat, stir in the cayenne and simmer for about 5 minutes or until steaming. Serve topped with the roasted corn.

TIPS: Most soups taste better the day after they are prepared. So, make enough for leftovers, cool thoroughly and refrigerate.

PREP TIME: *1 hour*
YIELD: *8 cups*
MAKES 4 TO 6 SERVINGS
NUTRITION TOTALS: *Calories 107.6, Fat .83g, Protein 2.2g, Carbohydrate 23.65g*

HOMEMADE CHICKEN STOCK: *1 cup = 39/1.4g/4.9g/0.9g*

Tomato-Basil Soup

This is a simple, delightful soup that goes well with a sandwich or salad.

Nonfat oil spray
1 medium onion, diced
6 large, vine-ripened tomatoes, diced
4 cups water
3 tablespoons powdered chicken stock
2 tablespoons pine nuts, roasted
¼ cup fresh basil, julienned
2 medium cloves garlic
2 tablespoons grated Parmesan cheese
1 tablespoon tomato paste
Salt and freshly ground pepper to taste

Options:
Toasted French bread slices

Preheat oven to 350 degrees. In a large soup pot generously sprayed with oil, sauté the onion over medium heat until translucent. Add the tomatoes and cook for five minutes. Mix in water and powdered stock and simmer for twenty minutes. Meanwhile, roast the pine nuts in the oven for about three minutes or until golden. Watch them carefully to avoid burning. Remove the nuts and set aside to cool. In a food processor or blender, pulse the basil, garlic, Parmesan, tomato paste and cooled pine nuts until creamy. Stir the mixture into the hot soup and cook for another 2 minutes. Add salt and pepper to taste and serve sprinkled with a little extra Parmesan. Freshly toasted French bread slices are excellent for dipping.

PREP TIME: *30 minutes*
YIELD: *9 cups*
MAKES 4½ SERVINGS
NUTRITION TOTALS: *Calories 107, Fat 3.1g, Protein: 4.2g, Carbohydrate 16.5g*
FRENCH BREAD: *1 slice = 81/1.1g/2.7g/14.8g*

Potato-Spinach Soup

With its deep potato-spinach flavor, this soup is hearty and very comforting to eat.

Nonfat oil spray
2 medium leeks, white part only, washed and thinly sliced
2 cups water
3 tablespoons powdered chicken stock
3 medium potatoes, peeled, quartered, rinsed
1 pound spinach, rinsed, stalks removed, julienned
2 tablespoons fresh dill, chopped
2 teaspoons Old Bay seasoning
½ teaspoon ground nutmeg
1 cup skinned, diced tomato
Salt to taste

In a large soup pot generously sprayed with oil, sauté the leeks over medium heat until they are translucent. Add the water and chicken stock powder and bring to a boil. Add the potatoes and simmer on low heat until they are tender. Remove the leeks and potatoes, drain and set aside to cool. Reserve the broth. Puree the cooked vegetables until smooth and return mixture to broth. Stir in spinach, dill and spices, and simmer for another 5 minutes or until spinach cooks down. Adjust salt to taste and serve garnished with diced tomatoes.

PREP TIME: *1 hour*
YIELD: *8 cups*
Makes 4 servings
NUTRITION TOTALS: *Calories 106, Fat .75g, Protein 5.25g, Carbohydrate 29.25g*

Smoked Turkey Sandwich

A strongly flavored, satisfying combination of sweet mustard, mild turkey and cheese. This sandwich can become a lunchtime staple.

1 tablespoon nonfat honey mustard
1 tablespoon cranberry sauce
½ tablespoon finely chopped fresh sage
2 slices multigrain bread, toasted
4 ounces shaved smoked turkey breast
1 leaf green leaf lettuce
1 slice fresh tomato
1 slice low fat Swiss cheese

Option:

½ to ¼ tablespoon chopped hot pepper (long red hot, jalapeño, Scotch bonnet, habanero)

In a medium bowl, combine the mustard, cranberry sauce and sage. Spread it on the toast and build a sandwich with the remaining ingredients. To spice it up, mix your favorite hot pepper into the mustard spread (handle fresh hot pepper carefully; avoid contact with eyes).

TIPS: Take caution chopping fresh hot pepper. Wear surgical plastic gloves (or cover hands with sandwich bags) and avoid touching eyes with fingers that have come in contact with pepper.

PREP TIME: *10 minutes*
YIELD: *1 sandwich*
MAKES 1 SERVING
NUTRITION TOTALS: *Calories 366. Fat 7.8g, Protein 23.8g, Carbohydrate 54.5g; hot pepper 3/0g/0.3g/1.0g*

Vegetarian Pita Pocket

This colorful, multitextured sandwich has a pleasant tang and makes for a healthy lunchtime treat.

3 tablespoons plain yogurt
2 teaspoons chopped fresh tarragon
1 teaspoon Dijon mustard
8 spinach leaves, rinsed and trimmed
4 medium mushrooms, thinly sliced
4 asparagus spears, rinsed, trimmed and blanched
2 slices medium tomato
½ medium cucumber, peeled and thinly sliced
½ small avocado, sliced crosswise
2 tablespoons raisins
Pinch salt and freshly ground black pepper
1 whole wheat pita
Options:
Mixed fruits
Grilled vegetables
1 tablespoon balsamic vinegar
1 tablespoon freshly chopped herbs

In a medium bowl, mix yogurt, mustard and tarragon. Toss in the remaining ingredients, except the pita, and adjust the seasoning to taste. Fill half of a lightly warmed pita with half of the prepared mixture, or 1 ½ cups of a grilled vegetable medley. Add all vegetables and toss gently. Season with salt and pepper. Fill pita halves with vegetable mixture, being sure to distribute mixture evenly. A small bowl of mixed fresh fruit is a classic accompaniment to this meal.

Recipes

PREP TIME: *25 minutes*
YIELD: *2 filled pita halves*
MAKES 2 SERVINGS
NUTRITION TOTALS: *Calories 182, Fat 8.6g, Protein 6.9g, Carbohydrate 28.9g*

GRILLED VEGETABLES: *½ cup = 13/0.1g/0.8g/2.8g*

BALSAMIC VINEGAR: *1 T= 2/0g/0.1g/.8g*

HERBS: *average, 1 T fresh, chopped = 2/0g/0.1g/0.3g*

Cold Crisp Penne Salad with Tangy Grilled Chicken and Vegetables

A wonderful array of tastes and textures makes this a very special lunch. This salad takes a little effort to prepare but it is truly worth the effort.

Marinade

    4 tablespoons lemon juice, fresh squeezed or commercial
    2 cloves garlic
    1 medium shallot, peeled
    1 tablespoon chopped fresh cilantro
    1 tablespoon chopped fresh basil
    1 teaspoon chopped fresh thyme
    ½ to 1 teaspoon chopped jalapeno pepper

For the grill

    2 boneless, skinless chicken breasts
    1 small red pepper, deseeded and cut in half
    1 small eggplant, cut lengthwise into ½-inch-thick slices
    ¼ cup oil for brushing grill, chicken and vegetables

Tomato vinaigrette

    ¼ cup sundried tomatoes
    ¼ cup red-wine vinegar
    1 medium shallot, sliced
    2 tablespoons coarsely chopped fresh basil
    1 tablespoon coarsely chopped fresh cilantro
    2 anchovy fillets
    1 ½ teaspoons paprika
    ½ cup olive oil
    Freshly ground black pepper

For the salad bowl
    4 ounces penne pasta (1 ¼ cups cooked)
    6 cups coarsely chopped romaine lettuce
    5 cherry tomatoes, halved
    ¼ cup grated Parmesan cheese
    ¼ cup toasted, chopped walnuts

In a food processor or blender, pulse the marinade ingredients to a fine mince. Toss the chicken breasts with the marinade in a shallow bowl, cover and set aside for about one hour. Cook the penne al dente, drain, rinse in cold water and set aside to cool. Trim and cut the pepper and eggplant.

While the grill preheats, prepare the romaine and cherry tomatoes and make the vinaigrette. Soften sundried tomatoes in the vinegar for about 5 minutes in a small bowl. In a food processor or blender, pulse the tomato-vinegar mixture to a smooth paste with the rest of the dressing ingredients, except the oil. Slowly add the oil while pulsing for 1 minute more. Adjust the seasoning and set aside.

Lightly brush the chicken and vegetables with oil before grilling. Discard the marinade. Grill the chicken about 5 minutes on each side; vegetables about 3 minutes on each side. Remove them from the grill and let cool. Julienne the chicken and vegetables and gently combine them in a large bowl with salad ingredients and penne. Toss the salad with the vinaigrette. Serve sprinkled with Parmesan and walnuts.

TIPS: Soak greens in ice for extra crispness. Refrigerated dressing keeps for up to one week.

Chicken may be grilled on the broiler setting in a home oven, but the rich charcoal character will be lost. This dish also makes a wonderful dinner entree.

PREP TIME: *40 minutes*
YIELD:

> *chicken = 2 ½ cups*
> *vegetables = 1 cup*
> *penne = 2 ½ cups*

Makes 2–3 servings

NUTRITION TOTALS: *Calories 474, Fat 5.6g, Protein 60.7g, Carbohydrate:50.1g*

MARINADE
PREP TIME: *15 minutes*
YIELD: *¾ cups*
NUTRITION TOTALS: *Calories 44.5, Fat .67g, Protein1.2g, Carbohydrate 30.97g*

VINAIGRETTE
PREP TIME: *20 minutes*
YIELD: *¾ cups*
NUTRITION TOTALS: *Calories 271, Fat 27.5g, Protein 2.3g, Carbohydrate 5.2g*

SALAD GREENS
PREP TIME: *8 minutes*
YIELD: *8 cups*
NUTRITION TOTALS: *Calories 21, Fat .6g, Protein 3.0g, Carbohydrate 4.2g*

Dinner

MENU 1
Pan-Seared Ginger Snapper with Pineapple Sauce
and Spicy Pepper Polenta
Garden salad
Lemonade or herbal tea mixture (8 oz.)

MENU 2
Roast Turkey Breast
Cornbread Stuffing
Sour Cream–Carrot Mashed Sweet Potatoes
Ice water with lemon (8 oz.)

MENU 3
Barbecue Chicken Sandwich
Mixed Green Salad with Orange-Ginger Dressing
Low-sugar lemonade (8 oz.)

MENU 4
Chicken-Stuffed Eggplant
Couscous
Garden salad
Mint iced tea (8 oz.)

Pan-Seared Ginger Snapper with Pineapple Sauce and Spicy Pepper Polenta

This dinner not only is a tart, crisp, spicy way to add excitement to the evening meal; it looks like a painting on a plate.

4 6-ounce red snapper filets or similar fish, such as striped bass
1 tablespoon finely grated ginger
1 tablespoon finely chopped fresh cilantro
1 tablespoon finely chopped basil
1 clove garlic, minced
2 tablespoons lemon juice, fresh or bottled
Salt and freshly ground black pepper to taste
Nonfat oil spray
½ cup flour for sprinkling

Spicy Pepper Polenta
1 ½ cups low fat chicken stock or water
½ cup coarse ground cornmeal
Nonfat oil spray
¼ cup finely diced red pepper
¼ cup finely diced green pepper
¼ teaspoon red pepper flakes

Pineapple Sauce:
1 cup pureed pineapple
2 tablespoons lemon juice, fresh or bottled
2 tablespoons low salt soy sauce
12 fresh snow pea pods

Preheat oven to 400 degrees. In a shallow bowl, marinate the fish in the combined herbs, garlic and lemon juice for about 1 hour, covered with plastic wrap. (Almost any type of nonoily, flaky fish does well in this recipe.)

Meanwhile, in a medium-size saucepan, mix chicken stock and cornmeal. Bring it to a boil, then reduce the heat and cook for about 15 minutes, continually stirring. Sauté the peppers in a well-sprayed small pan for about 2 minutes. Add the red pepper flakes. Stir the pepper blend into the polenta and cook an additional 5 minutes. Spread the polenta evenly in a greased, 8x8-inch pan and let it cool thoroughly until firm. Slice the polenta into diamonds and grill them lightly on both sides in a hot, well-greased medium frying pan. Set diamonds aside on a warm plate.

Spray a large frying pan with nonfat oil spray, and briefly place on medium heat. Sprinkle the fish filets with flour and fry on one side for 5 minutes or until a light golden color. Flip fish over into a lightly greased ovenproof baking dish and finish cooking in the oven for about 6 minutes, or until cooked through.

In a small saucepan, combine the pineapple puree, lemon juice and soy sauce. Simmer over high heat for five minutes, add snow pea pods and set aside. (The snow pea pods will cook briefly but will retain crispness.)

Onto each of four warmed plates, spoon out a quarter of the pineapple sauce, fan out a quarter of the snow peas, and lay a fish fillet in the center with a grilled polenta diamond on both sides. Serve immediately.

FISH
PREP TIME: *1 hour, 40 minutes*
YIELD: *24 oz. fish; 1 ¼ cup marinade*
NUTRITION TOTALS: *Calories 254, Fat 3.35g, Protein 46.1g, Carbohydrate 8.1g*

POLENTA
PREP TIME: *20 minutes*
YIELD: *4 cups*

NUTRITION TOTALS: *Calories 126, Fat 1.6g, Protein 3.4g, Carbohydrate 26.2g*

PINEAPPLE SAUCE

PREP TIME: *8 minutes*

YIELD: *2 cups*

NUTRITION TOTALS: *Calories 65, Fat .3g, Protein 2.05g, Carbohydrate 12.6g*

Roast Turkey Breast with Corn Bread Stuffing and Sweet Potatoes

This is a beautiful, tender turkey breast that is infused with a sweet fruit flavor. The entire dish requires a minimum of effort and delivers maximum results.

1 4- to 5-pound boneless turkey breast
1 medium onion, peeled and sliced
1 medium apple, cored, sliced and seeded
1 medium orange, sliced and seeded
1 stalk celery, cut in 4 pieces
2 cloves garlic, crushed
2 tablespoons chopped fresh sage
2 teaspoons Old Bay seasoning

Preheat oven to 400 degrees. Lay enough aluminum foil across a roasting dish so that there is enough to wrap the turkey breast completely. Place all the vegetables, fruits and seasonings on the foil, then lay the breast on top of them. Wrap the foil loosely around the breast, securing all seams tightly. Bake for 1 hour. Check for doneness with a meat thermometer, which should register 180 degrees, or pierce a side with a knife. The turkey is ready when the juices run clear. Continue cooking for about 15 minutes, then remove turkey to a warm serving platter, cover and let rest for about 15 minutes.

TIPS: The reserved pan juices may be turned into a light gravy by stirring in a mixture of 2 teaspoons cornstarch and ¼ cup warm water.

PREP TIME: *1 ½ hours*
YIELD: *1 5-pound turkey breast*
MAKES 6 SERVINGS
NUTRITION TOTALS: *Per 7-ounce serving: Calories 314, Fat 6.4g, Protein 39.8g, Carbohydrate 0g*

Cornbread Stuffing

The perfect partner to a turkey dinner. Great for holidays or everyday.

Nonfat oil spray
4 strips turkey bacon
½ cup coarsely chopped onion
½ cup coarsely chopped celery
½ cup peeled, cored and coarsely chopped Granny Smith apple
2 cloves garlic, chopped
½ cup chopped, roasted and peeled chestnuts
2 cups corn muffin crumbs
3 tablespoons chopped fresh parsley
2 tablespoons chopped fresh sage
2 tablespoons chopped fresh thyme
¼ cup raisins
1 cup low fat chicken stock
Freshly ground black pepper to taste

Preheat oven to 350 degrees. While the turkey is roasting, sauté the turkey bacon in a lightly oiled fry pan for 2 minutes. Add the onion, celery and garlic and cook for another 5 minutes. Remove the mixture from the heat and cool. In a food processor, pulse the cooled mixture to a fine texture. Pour it into a large bowl and add the rest of the ingredients, combining them thoroughly. Season to taste. Spread the stuffing into a lightly oiled, 10-inch baking dish and bake for about 20 minutes.

PREP TIME: *30 minutes*
YIELD: *8 cups*
MAKES 4 TO 6 SERVINGS
NUTRITION TOTALS: *Calories 91.2, Fat 1.15g, Protein 3.05g, Carbohydrate 14.7g*

Sour Cream–Carrot Mashed Sweet Potatoes

The final complement to a wonderful meal is this sweet potato delight.

2 large sweet potatoes
2 carrots, peeled
Pinch of cinnamon
¼ cup low fat sour cream
2 tablespoons orange marmalade

In a large pot of boiling water, cook potatoes and carrots for about 20 minutes, or until fork tender. Remove the vegetables from the hot water and set aside to cool. Peel the cooled potatoes and mash them in a large bowl with the carrots, marmalade and cinnamon. Whip in sour cream with a wire whisk until well combined.

TIPS: An electric mixer or food processor produces a lighter mashed potato with more volume and a delicate texture. Retain nutrients by cooking whole potatoes with skins on.

PREP TIME: *40 minutes*
YIELD: *3 cups*
MAKES 3 SERVINGS
NUTRITION TOTALS: *Calories 131, Fat .58g, Protein 2.1g, Carbohydrate 31.1g*

Barbecue Chicken Sandwich

A delicious, nutritious, easy-to-make dinner for people on the go.

2 boneless, skinless chicken breasts
2 whole wheat Kaiser rolls, sliced in half
2 romaine lettuce leaves
2 slices tomato
2 thin slices red onion

Marinade
Nonfat oil spray
½ cup chopped onion
1 clove garlic, chopped
1 cup ketchup
½ cup crushed or pureed pineapple
2 tablespoons Worcestershire sauce
2 tablespoons packed dark brown sugar
2 tablespoons cider vinegar
1 tablespoon mustard

Option:
¼ small hot pepper, finely chopped (jalapeño, Scotch bonnet)

Preheat the oven to 400 degrees. In a lightly oiled fry pan over medium heat, sauté the onion and garlic until translucent. Add the remaining marinade ingredients and simmer on low heat for about 15 minutes. Meanwhile, grill chicken breasts for about 3 minutes on both sides. Remove the chicken to a shallow baking dish, pour over the marinade, cover and let sit for 30 minutes. Bake the chicken in the oven for 5 minutes.

On toasted Kaiser rolls, build sandwiches with equal amounts of chicken, lettuce, tomato and onion.

TIP: Take caution chopping fresh hot pepper. Wear surgical plastic gloves (or cover hands with sandwich bags) and avoid touching eyes with fingers that have come in contact with pepper.

PREP TIME: *40 minutes*
YIELD: *2 sandwiches*
MAKES 2 SERVINGS
NUTRITION TOTALS: *Calories 502, Fat 5.1g, Protein 56.9g, Carbohydrate 55.4g*

Mixed Green Salad with Orange-Ginger Dressing

The perfect complement to any sandwich.

> 6 oz. mixed greens (any combination of red leaf, romaine and Bibb
> lettuce; radicchio, spinach, frisee, arugula)
> ¾ cup peeled, sliced cucumber
> 1 medium tomato, cut into 6 wedges
> 1 orange, peeled, seeded and sectioned into wedges

Ginger Dressing:
> ¾ cup orange juice
> ¼ cup rice wine vinegar
> 2 teaspoons Dijon mustard
> 1 teaspoon minced fresh ginger
> 1 teaspoon honey
> 1 teaspoon low-salt soy sauce
> 1 garlic clove, minced

Combine all the dressing ingredients in a pourable, sealable container and set aside. In a large salad bowl, mix the greens with the cucumber and tomato and gently toss with dressing to coat. Serve garnished with orange wedges.

PREP TIME: *20 minutes*
YIELD: *6 ¾ cups*
MAKES 2 TO 3 SERVINGS
NUTRITION TOTALS: *Calories 106, Fat 1g, Protein 2.1g, Carbohydrate 21.3g*

Chicken-Stuffed Eggplant

This tender, casserole-style dish just melts in your mouth. One of my all-time favorites!

4 medium eggplants, cut lengthwise into ¼-inch slices
1 ½ pounds ground skinless and boneless chicken breast
1 tablespoon olive oil
1 egg
2 egg whites
1 medium onion, finely chopped
1 tablespoon finely chopped parsley
Nonfat oil spray
1 large (27.7 ounce) jar tomato sauce
½ cup grated Parmesan cheese
Salt and freshly ground pepper to taste

Options:

½ cup pine nuts
8 cups cooked couscous

Preheat oven to 400 degrees. Bake eggplant on cookie sheets sprayed with nonfat oil spray in oven for about 10 minutes or until tender but not crisp. Let them cool before handling. Meanwhile thoroughly combine the chicken with a tablespoon of oil, egg, egg whites, onion and parsley. Adjust seasoning. Place a generous tablespoon of filling on each eggplant strip, roll it up and set it seam-side down in a lightly sprayed 13 x 9 x 2-inch baking dish. Pour the sauce over the rolls, sprinkle the top with Parmesan and bake for 15 to 20 minutes, or until thoroughly cooked through.

PREP TIME: *1 hour*
YIELD: *30 rolls; will vary with size of eggplant strips*
MAKES 4 TO 6 SERVINGS
NUTRITION TOTALS: *Per 6-roll serving: Calories 189, Fat 6.12g, Protein 26.4g, Carbohydrate 14.82g*

Snacks

Raw vegetables (you can use salsa or teriyaki sauce
as a topping)

Fruits

Fruit juice (orange and grapefruit are my top picks)

Nonfat pretzels (one to one-and-a-half oz.)

Low fat, air-popped popcorn (you can top with salsa,
Worcestershire sauce, vinegar or black or cayenne pepper)

Rice cakes (try the plain with fruit on top)

Soup (noncream base)

Baked potato (topped with salsa, Worcestershire sauce or other low
fat topping)

Brown rice

Low fat frozen yogurt

Low fat frozen yogurt bars

Low fat/low sugar frozen fruit bars

Low fat cookies

TIPS: A good snack should be about 80 to 150 calories. Adjust your servings accordingly. Herbal or mint tea is also an excellent no-calorie snack and can be enjoyed with any other snack.